SOMATIC WORKOUTS

For Seniors Over 60

Gentle Exercises To Relieve Pain, Reduce Stress, And Restore Flexibility

DR. HAMRICK NELSON

Disclaimer

The information and exercises in this book, Somatic Workouts for Seniors Over 60, are intended to support your journey toward improved mobility, flexibility, and overall well-being. However, they are not substitutes for professional medical advice, diagnosis, or treatment.

Before beginning any new exercise program, including the somatic workouts described in this book, it is important to consult with your healthcare provider or a licensed medical professional, particularly if you have pre-existing conditions, injuries, or other health concerns.

The exercises outlined here are designed to be gentle and adaptable, but every individual is unique. Listening to your body and proceeding at a pace that feels comfortable for you is essential. If you experience discomfort, pain, or unexpected symptoms while performing the exercises, please stop immediately and seek professional guidance.

This book is intended to educate and inspire, providing general guidance for seniors who want to enhance their quality of life through mindful movement. By engaging in the exercises described, you acknowledge that you are doing so voluntarily and at your own risk.

Your safety and well-being are my priority, and I encourage you to approach this journey with care, curiosity, and professional support when needed.

Table of Contents

ABOUT THE AUTHOR

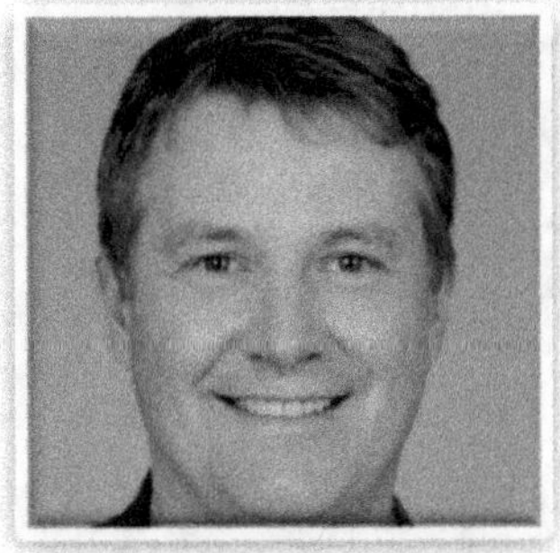 Dr. Hamrick Nelson is a leading voice in fitness and wellness, with a deep passion for helping individuals of all ages live healthier, more active lives. With over two decades of experience in the health and fitness industry, Dr. Nelson has dedicated his career to promoting accessible exercise routines for people at every stage of life. His approach is rooted in the belief that movement is for everyone, regardless of age or physical limitations.

Through his extensive research and hands-on experience, he understands the unique challenges faced by individuals of different ages, and he's made it his mission to help them maintain their independence, strength, and vitality. He combines practical knowledge with compassion, creating tailored fitness programs that prioritize safety and long-term health benefits.

Holding advanced degrees in physical therapy and exercise science, Dr. Nelson has worked with countless individuals to enhance their mobility, flexibility, and overall well-being. His books, workshops, and speaking engagements reflect his commitment to helping people of all ages, whether young or senior, stay fit, feel strong, and live life to the fullest.

INTRODUCTION

The path to better health, particularly in our later years, is deeply personal and frequently laden with problems we never anticipated. I've had the pleasure of dealing with innumerable people over the years who have sought relief from chronic pain, stiffness, and stress, often feeling as if their finest years were behind them. This book, **"Somatic Workouts for Seniors Over 60,"** is for people like them, and maybe even you. It is a guide not just to recovering bodily ease, but also to regaining joy, peace, and confidence in movement.

Let me start with a story.

*Several years ago, on a speaking engagement in Manchester, I met an intriguing woman named Hannah Caldwell. Hannah was 66 at the time, a retired librarian with a sharp wit and a fascinating personality. She'd come to my mindful movement session not because she thought it would benefit her, but because, as she expressed it, **"I've already tried everything else."***

Hannah's narrative was about quiet resilience. For years, she had suffered from persistent neck and shoulder discomfort, the result of decades spent slumped over desks and computers. The agony had gotten so bad that even simple chores like reading a book or raising a teacup became impossible. But it wasn't just the physical anguish that held her down; it was also the mental cost.

"Every time I struggle to tie my shoes or carry groceries," she told me during a break, "I feel like I'm losing a part of myself. "It feels like my body is betraying me."

I could see the frustration in her eyes, but what struck me the most was her drive to take action. Despite her reservations, she came to my session because she was determined to succeed. And that led her to somatic movement practices.

And this is the turning point.

Hannah was suspicious at first, as are many others. Somatic activities don't resemble traditional workouts. They don't involve pushing your body to its limits or breaking a sweat. Instead, they entail slow, purposeful motions that aim to integrate your mind and body, allowing you to listen to the messages your body is sending and respond in a way that promotes healing.

During the first session, I led Hannah and the other participants through a basic somatic exercise that blended shoulder rolls with conscious breathing. It's a technique for relieving tension and increasing upper-body mobility. Hannah moved stiffly at first, only twisting her shoulders slightly. However, as we progressed, I saw her movements become smoother and fluid.

Hannah approached me after the session, her expression full of inquiry and hope. "That was... different," she replied, hesitating to find the appropriate words. "I don't feel as constricted now. It's subtle, but it's present."

Hannah continued to practice the exercises every day for the next three weeks. Each time we called, she mentioned tiny wins like waking up without stiffness, taking a pain-free walk in her garden, or finally being able to knit for more than a few minutes at a time.

*Six months later, Hannah mailed me a handwritten note. It started with a simple yet profound statement: **"YOU'VE GIVEN ME MY LIFE BACK."***

Hannah's experience is just one of several that inspired this book. Somatic workouts are not a miracle treatment; they will not eliminate all of your pain overnight or return you to your twenties. However, they are transformative in their way. They provide a peaceful, approachable, yet deeply empowering approach to healing.

For seniors over 60, the challenges of aging might feel like an uphill climb. Stiffness appears where there was once flexibility. Pain becomes an unpleasant friend. Stress, worry, and the emotional impact of these bodily changes can be significant. Somatic workouts address all of these issues without fighting your body, but rather by working with it—respecting its needs and potential for growth and restoration.

This book is designed to walk you through every stage of the process, from comprehending the concepts of somatic movement to creating a personalized program that fits into your lifestyle. It's intended to be both practical and powerful, with workouts that are simple to follow and tailored to your specific needs.

In the following chapters, you will learn how somatic exercises can alleviate pain, reduce stress, and increase flexibility.

- The science behind somatic movement, including how it retrains the nervous system to promote better posture and mobility.
- Step-by-step exercises for several body areas, including the neck and shoulders, lower back, hips, and legs.
- Breathing techniques for relaxing your mind and boosting your body's natural healing processes.

- Tips for developing a daily regimen that suits your lifestyle and allows you to sustain your success over time.

Beyond the practicalities, this book is an invitation, an opportunity to reconnect with your body in a way that feels caring rather than punishing. It's about regaining the joy of movement and the confidence that comes with knowing you can care for yourself, regardless of your age or physical condition.

If you've read this book, I'm guessing you'll recognize some of yourself in Hannah's story, or in the tales of countless others who have traveled this journey. Perhaps you've experienced the frustration of limited movement, the aching of chronic pain, or the burden of stress and anxiety. You are not alone.

The exercises and techniques in this book have been tested and perfected over years of use with people from many walks of life, including the elderly who feared they'd never be able to move freely again. Their triumphs, like Hannah's, demonstrate the power of somatic movement.

Before you begin the activities, I invite you to reflect on why you chose this path. What do you want to achieve? Is it pain relief, increased flexibility, or simply the ability to conduct your favorite hobbies without strain? Write down your objectives and keep them close as you progress through the chapters.

Remember that growth isn't about perfection. It's about taking tiny, persistent steps towards the life you want to live. And, along the way, be kind to yourself. Celebrate your accomplishments, no matter how minor, and tackle problems with patience and inquiry.

This is the time to recover your health, peace of mind, and vigor. You, like Hannah, have the strength and commitment to make significant changes. Allow this book to be your guide, companion, and source of inspiration as you embark on this adventure.

Welcome to "Somatic Workouts for Seniors Over 60". Let's get started.

CHAPTER 1: UNDERSTANDING SOMATIC WORKOUTS FOR SENIORS

What Is Somatic Movement?

Somatic movement is a type of massage and exercise that stresses awareness, mindfulness, and the relationship between mind and body. This movement technique, based on somatic principles, teaches people how to detect and regulate their body's movements more consciously and intentionally. Somatic movement can be a transforming technique for seniors, particularly those over the age of 60, to improve flexibility, reduce pain, and promote mental well-being.

Somatic movement can be traced back to the broader discipline of somatics, which emerged in the mid-twentieth century in response to a growing interest in alternative approaches to health and wellbeing, as well as bodily awareness. Thomas Hanna, philosopher and movement educator, created the word "somatics" in the 1970s. Hanna defined somatics as a discipline that emphasizes the lived experience of the body—how we perceive, feel, and move from within—rather than considering the body as a mechanical structure.

Hanna's work expanded on the pioneering work of earlier practitioners, such as Moshe Feldenkrais, who created the Feldenkrais Method, a technique that stresses movement and awareness to improve function and reduce pain. Similarly, Ida Rolf developed Rolfing, a method for realigning the body's structure to improve movement and reduce tension. F. also had a considerable influence. M. Alexander invented the Alexander Technique, which focuses on releasing habitual tension patterns to improve posture and performance.

These pioneers recognized the intrinsic link between the body and mind, questioning the traditional distinction between physical and mental health. They looked into how regular movement patterns, posture, and even emotional stress could affect physical well-being and cause tension or pain in the body.

Hanna elaborated on these ideas, stressing the nervous system's function in managing movement and tension. He coined the term "sensory-motor amnesia," a syndrome in which the brain loses the ability to appropriately feel and regulate specific muscles as a result of chronic stress, injury, or bad habits. Individuals can retrain their nervous systems to release tension, improve posture, and restore functional mobility by engaging in somatic movement activities.

The somatic movement has grown into a multifaceted discipline that includes methods such as Body-Mind Centering (created by Bonnie Bainbridge Cohen), the Rosen Method, and the Continuum Movement. These practices all aim to promote better awareness, ease, and harmony in the body through intentional, conscious movement. Somatic movement is now widely used in therapeutic, fitness, and wellness settings, providing an opportunity for people of all ages, including elders, to improve their physical and emotional health.

Principles Of Somatic Movement

1. Mind-Body Connection: At the heart of somatic movement is the concept of connecting the mind and body. This relationship is important since many people, particularly as they age, lose awareness of their body's sensations. For example, we may unintentionally acquire bad posture or movement habits that cause pain or discomfort. Somatic movement entails paying attention to these feelings and becoming aware of habitual patterns of tension, discomfort, or immobility. Once identified, these habits can be gradually corrected, resulting in greater posture, mobility, and pain relief.

2. Awareness through Movement: Somatic movement emphasizes the internal feeling of movement over exterior achievements such as strength or endurance. It's not about how far you can stretch or how fast you can move; it's about feeling what's going on in your body as you move. Slowing down activities and paying close attention to physiological sensations can help people release tension, develop flexibility, and gain a better understanding of their bodies.

3. Role of the Nervous System: One important feature of somatic movement is its effect on the neurological system.

Our brain and nervous system influence how we move and react to external stimuli. Over time, the brain can acquire habits in the body's movement patterns, known as "muscle memory." In some situations, poor posture or misuse of specific muscles can result in pain and dysfunction. Somatic exercises retrain the neural system, allowing the body to develop healthier and more efficient movement patterns.

4. Slowness and intentionality: Unlike high-impact exercises or many traditional stretching routines, somatic movement is usually slow, deliberate, and intentional. This is especially useful for elders with restricted mobility or chronic pain concerns. The goal is to perform motions softly and deliberately, allowing the body to release long-held tension and improve general function while avoiding harm. The movements are performed at a pace that allows the nervous system to reset and learn new, pain-free patterns.

Benefits Of Somatic Movement For Seniors

Somatic movement offers a comprehensive and gentle approach to treating the specific difficulties that elders confront, such as pain, stiffness, and emotional stress. Its benefits go beyond physical health, promoting cerebral clarity and emotional balance as well. *Here's a closer look at how it can improve the lives of elders:*

1. Chronic Pain Relief: Many seniors suffer from chronic discomfort in their neck, back, shoulders, and hips as a result of years of bad posture, injury, or misuse. Somatic exercises target these areas by relieving muscle tension and retraining the body to move more efficiently. This non-invasive, drug-free strategy helps elders manage their pain more effectively over time.

2. Enhanced Flexibility and Mobility: Flexibility frequently declines with age, limiting range of motion and making daily activities more challenging. Slow, deliberate movements promote joint flexibility and muscular suppleness over time, helping elders restore confidence in their ability to move comfortably.

3. Improved Balance and Fall Prevention: Falls are the biggest cause of injury among the elderly. Somatic

activity promotes balance by raising awareness of body alignment and spatial orientation. Moderate exercises strengthen core muscles and enhance coordination, making elders more stable and minimizing their risk of falling.

4. Stress and Anxiety Reduction: The mindfulness component of somatic movement helps to soothe the nervous system and induce relaxation. Breathing methods and slow, deliberate motions engage the parasympathetic nervous system, which is the body's "rest and digest" mode, reducing tension and anxiety.

5. Better Posture: Poor posture frequently causes discomfort, and pain, as well as respiratory and circulation problems. Somatic activities teach elders how to identify and correct postural misalignments. They can benefit from improved posture, increased mobility, and less strain on their shoulders, neck, and back by rebalancing muscle use and joint alignment.

6. Increased Self-Awareness: The somatic movement emphasizes becoming more aware of how the body feels and moves. This increased self-awareness enables elders to notice and resolve patterns of stress or strain,

thereby avoiding the development of chronic pain and stiffness over time.

7. Emotional Resilience and Mental Clarity: Somatic movement strengthens the mind-body connection, which promotes emotional well-being and mental clarity. Seniors who apply these approaches frequently report feeling more grounded, focused, and emotionally balanced. The moderate emphasis on movement also encourages relaxation, improves sleep quality, and alleviates symptoms of despair or anxiety.

8. Accessibility and Ease of Practice: Somatic exercises are adjustable to various levels of fitness and mobility, making them ideal for seniors, particularly those with physical disabilities. Movements can be performed seated, standing, or lying down, with no extra equipment necessary. This accessibility enables anyone to benefit, regardless of their current physical state.

Seniors who incorporate somatic movement into their daily routines might experience a restored sense of vigor, confidence, and independence, which improves their overall quality of life.

Somatic movement provides a comprehensive and gentle approach to enhancing seniors' physical and mental well-being. Somatic exercises, which focus on awareness, intention, and the mind-body connection, can help relieve pain, increase flexibility, and reduce stress. Somatic movement is a beneficial technique for seniors who want to stay active, ease discomfort, and reconnect with their bodies. It improves long-term health, vitality, and well-being.

How Somatic Movement Differs From Traditional Exercise

Somatic movement and traditional exercise serve distinct roles and approaches to physical activity. Traditional exercise focuses on developing strength, endurance, and physical performance through repetitive and frequently externally guided activities, whereas somatic movement stresses internal awareness, mindfulness, and the neuromuscular connection between the body and brain. Understanding these main characteristics can assist individuals in determining the best method for their objectives and circumstances, particularly for seniors or those suffering from chronic pain, stress, or mobility constraints.

1. Focus: Internal Awareness vs. External Performance

- Somatic Movement: The major purpose of somatic movement is to gain an internal understanding of how the body feels and moves. Practitioners are asked to concentrate on the feelings in their muscles, joints, and total body alignment while performing each movement. This internal attention helps to retrain the nervous system, relieve stress, and increase movement efficiency. Somatic movement is sometimes described as a personal journey of discovering and comprehending the body.

- Traditional Exercises: Traditional exercise often focuses on external performance measurements, such as how much weight can be lifted, how far one can run, or how many repetitions of a movement can be performed. The goal is frequently to produce measurable outcomes such as muscle increase, fat loss, or enhanced athletic performance. This method frequently prioritizes meeting outward standards above awareness of internal experiences.

2. Intensity: Gentle and Relaxed vs. Rigorous and Challenging

- Somatic Movement: Somatic activities are purposely slow, soft, and relaxing. The emphasis is on moving with ease, minimizing strain, and allowing the body to release accumulated tension. This milder approach is especially good for elders, those recuperating from injury, and those suffering from chronic pain because it reduces the chance of more strain or discomfort. Movements are carried out within a comfortable range of motion to guarantee safety and effectiveness.

- Traditional Exercises: Traditional workouts frequently include high-intensity or intense activities intended to test the body. These could involve hard weightlifting, high-impact cardio, or endurance training. While these activities can improve strength and stamina, they may not be appropriate for people who have physical limitations or require a more restorative approach to movement.

3. Approach: Corrective and therapeutic vs. Competitive and Goal-oriented

- Somatic Movement: Somatic techniques are fundamentally healing and remedial. Retraining the neural system helps to treat problematic movement patterns, chronic tension, and postural abnormalities. The goal is not to achieve a specific degree of fitness, but to restore the body's natural capacity to move freely and easily. Every action is approached as a thoughtful investigation, to minimize pain and expand the range of motion.

- Traditional Exercises: The traditional approach is frequently competitive or goal-oriented, whether the objective is to reduce weight, grow muscle, or run faster. This can occasionally lead to a "no pain, no gain" mentality, in which people push themselves to their limits, risking injury or exacerbating existing problems.

4. Connection: Mind-Body Integration vs. Mechanical Execution

- Somatic Movement: Every exercise in somatic movement involves both the mind and the body. Practitioners are taught to be fully present, observing how their body reacts to each movement. This awareness helps to retrain the brain-body relationship, resolving long-term stress or poor movement habits. For example, someone practicing somatics may concentrate on how their lower back feels during a basic pelvic tilt, making modifications to release tension as needed.

- Traditional Exercises: Traditional workouts frequently emphasize the mechanical execution of activities, such as maintaining good form or completing a predetermined number of reps. While proper form is important, the emphasis is frequently placed on the exterior appearance of the movement rather than the internal sensations. For example, someone lifting weights may be focused on finishing their reps without paying heed to small signs from their body.

5. Neuroplasticity: Reprogramming The Nervous System vs. Repetition of Movements

- Somatic Movement: Somatic exercises activate the neural system and modify movement patterns. This process is based on the brain's neuroplasticity, or ability to generate new neural connections. Somatic movement trains the brain to let go of harmful patterns, such as persistent muscle tension, in favor of healthier, more efficient ways of moving.

- Traditional Exercises: Traditional workouts use repetition and consistency to develop muscle memory. While this can boost strength and endurance, it does not always address faulty movement patterns. If someone with poor posture does not pay attention to their body mechanics, they may unintentionally reinforce their posture concerns during repetitive strength training routines.

6. Impact: Restorative vs. Stress-Inducing

- Somatic Movement: Somatic techniques are naturally restorative, facilitating relaxation, stress reduction, and a state of calm. They frequently use breathwork and mindfulness practices to create a contemplative state.

This makes somatic movement an excellent choice for anyone trying to alleviate anxiety, increase sleep, or recuperate from physical or mental damage.

- Traditional Exercises: While typical workouts might relieve stress for some people, they frequently activate the body's fight-or-flight response, particularly during high-intensity sessions. This can be invigorating, but it may not be appropriate for people who prefer a more relaxing and restorative approach to movement.

7. Customization: Personalized Experience vs. One-Size-Fits-All

- Somatic Movement: Somatic practices are very individualized. Practitioners are urged to listen to their bodies and modify moves to suit their specific demands and comfort levels. There are no clear guidelines for how far to stretch or how many repetitions to perform; what counts most is how the body feels during the exercise.

- Traditional Exercises: Traditional exercise programs frequently take a one-size-fits-all approach, with predetermined sets, reps, and weight guidelines. While personal trainers or coaches may suggest alterations, the overall framework of these activities is less adaptable than somatic practices.

8. Outcomes: Holistic Wellness versus Physical Fitness

- Somatic Movement: Somatic movement produces holistic results, addressing both physical and emotional well-being. Pain alleviation, increased mobility, decreased tension, and a stronger sense of bodily connection are among the benefits. Somatics can be viewed as a long-term practice that promotes general health and quality of life.

- Traditional Exercises: Traditional exercise produces mostly physical results, such as enhanced strength, endurance, and cardiovascular fitness. While these are beneficial for overall health, they may not address more serious issues such as persistent tension, bad posture, or stress.

Somatic movement is a gentle, thoughtful alternative to traditional exercise that emphasizes internal awareness, therapeutic effects, and the mind-body connection. Traditional workouts stress external performance and measurable results, whereas somatics focuses on how the body feels and moves. This makes it an excellent alternative for the elderly, those recovering from an injury, or anybody looking for a restorative and comprehensive approach to physical activity. By adopting somatic movement, practitioners can build a stronger bond with their bodies, relieve pain and stress, and attain long-term wellness.

Common Somatic Practices

Somatic movement comprises a wide range of techniques and disciplines that emphasize awareness, slow movement, and the mind-body connection. These practices are based on mindfulness and neuroplasticity concepts, and they aim to help people improve their physical and mental health by retraining their nervous systems. The following are some of the most popular somatic practices, their distinct techniques, and how they contribute to enhanced movement, flexibility, and emotional resilience.

1. Hanna Somatics

Thomas Hanna developed Hanna Somatics, a movement-based approach that aims to retrain the brain to release chronic muscle tension. It focuses on "sensory-motor amnesia," which occurs when the nervous system forgets how to relax specific muscles as a result of repeated stress or trauma.

Core Techniques:

- Pandiculation: This is the gradual contraction and release of muscles, combined with attention, to reset the nervous system.

- Awareness Training: Encourages people to identify regions of tightness or discomfort while moving and intentionally release tension.
- Functional Integration: Movements that replicate daily activities to increase overall ease and efficiency.

Benefits:
- Relief from persistent discomfort caused by tight muscles.
- Improved posture and alignment.
- Greater ease in carrying out daily duties.

Suitable for: Seniors, anyone with chronic pain, and anyone who has muscle tension from stress or repetitive strain.

2. The Feldenkrais Method

Moshe Feldenkrais developed this method to improve movement patterns and posture through conscious, exploratory motions. It is predicated on the notion that increased body awareness leads to more efficient and pain-free movement.

Core Techniques:

- Awareness Through Movement (ATM): Guided sessions in which participants make modest, delicate motions while focusing on their interior sensations.
- Functional Integration (FI) is a one-on-one therapy in which a practitioner gently guides the individual's body through new movement possibilities.

Benefits:
- Improved coordination and balance.
- Reduced physical discomfort or stiffness.
- Improved understanding of habitual movement patterns and their effects on the body.

Suitable for: Seniors, sportsmen, dancers, and those recuperating from injuries or surgery.

3. Alexander Technique

The Alexander Technique aims to improve posture, alignment, and general movement efficiency. Created by F. M. Alexander, this approach is especially beneficial for relieving physical strain produced by bad posture and habitual tension.

Core Techniques:

- Postural Awareness: Teaching people to identify and release needless strain in their neck, shoulders, and back.
- Dynamic Movement: Promoting smooth, balanced motion in daily tasks like sitting, standing, and walking.
- Inhibition and Direction: Learning to pause before moving and deliberately guiding the body to act with less effort.

Benefits:
- Improved posture and spinal alignment.
- Reduced stress and tension in the body.
- Enhanced performance for musicians, actors, and other professionals who require precise movement.

Suitable for: Seniors with poor posture, those suffering from neck or back pain, and those looking for greater control over their movements.

4. Body-Mind Centering (BMC)

Bonnie Bainbridge Cohen created Body-Mind Centering, a holistic somatic technique that combines movement with an in-depth investigation of anatomy, physiology, and human developmental patterns.

Core Techniques:

- Bodily System Embodiment: Participants learn to perceive and manipulate various bodily systems, such as bones, muscles, and organs, which helps them become more self-aware.
- Developmental Movement Patterns are movements influenced by early childhood development that aim to restore natural body mechanics.
- Somatic Dialogue is the exploration of the body's emotional and energy relationships to aid healing.

Benefits:
- Increased coordination and fluidity in movement.
- Improved grasp of the body's anatomy and functions.
- Somatic exploration helps to improve emotional resilience.

Suitable for: Yoga, dance, and therapy practitioners, as well as elders looking for a stronger connection with their bodies.

5. Somatic Yoga

Somatic Yoga combines classic yoga postures with somatic concepts, emphasizing slow, focused movements and internal awareness. This practice invites practitioners to investigate their body's sensations and limitations without judgment.

Core Techniques:

- Gentle Yoga Poses: Designed to be accessible and safe for people of all ages and abilities.
- Mindful breathing is the practice of coordinating breath and movement to enhance calm and attention.
- Intentional Relaxation: releasing tension during and after poses to strengthen the mind-body connection.

Benefits:
- Increased flexibility and strength without exertion.
- Reduced anxiety and increased emotional well-being.
- Gentle treatment for injuries or persistent pain.

Suitable for: Seniors, beginners in yoga, and people with limited mobility.

6. Continuum Movement

Continuum Movement, created by Emilie Conrad, investigates the fluid nature of the body and its relationship to the natural rhythms of the planet. It promotes healing and vitality through breathing, sound, and gentle movements.

Core Techniques:

- Breath Awareness: Deep, expansive breathing that promotes calm and energy flow.
- Undulating Motions: Fluid, wave-like movements that resemble natural patterns observed in water and other organic systems.
- Sound Integration is the use of vocalizations to relieve tension and increase interior awareness.

Benefits:
- Increased vitality and energy.
- Improved range of motion and joint health.
- Emotional relief and reduced stress.

Suitable for: Seniors, dancers, and anyone seeking alternative therapeutic approaches.

7. Trager's Approach

The Trager Approach, developed by Dr. Milton Trager, emphasizes soft, rhythmic movements to relieve tension and promote a sensation of lightness and comfort in the body.

Core Techniques:

- Table Work: A practitioner gently rocks and moves the client's body while they lie on a massage table, encouraging relaxation.
- Mentastics: Self-care exercises that use gentle, joyful movements to incorporate the advantages of table work into everyday living.

Benefits:
- Relief from chronic pain and tension.
- Increased sense of freedom in movement.
- Reduced stress and increased overall well-being.

Suitable for: Individuals seeking stress alleviation, those healing from accidents, and senior citizens with mobility issues.

8. Eutony

Eutony, created by Gerda Alexander, focuses on developing harmony within the body by growing awareness of tension and releasing it via gentle movement and touch.

Core Techniques:

- Tactile awareness is the exploration of the body's texture, weight, and shape through touch.
- Movement Exploration: Gentle, flowing exercises that improve balance and fluidity.
- Relaxation Techniques: Ways to relieve stress and promote a sense of calm.

Benefits:
- Increased physical awareness and coordination.
- Reduced muscular stiffness and discomfort.
- Improved emotional equilibrium.

Suitable for: Seniors, people with chronic stress, and those looking for a meditative movement practice.

With so many somatic practices accessible, it's critical to select one that matches your objectives, physical condition, and interests. Each practice has distinct characteristics, and many may be tailored to meet specific needs. Whether you want to relieve chronic pain, improve your posture, or achieve a deeper sensation of relaxation, a somatic approach can help you reconnect with your body and move more freely.

Who Can Benefit From Somatic Movement?

Somatic movement is a diverse and inclusive approach to physical and mental well-being that provides significant advantages to people of all ages, physical abilities, and health issues. Its emphasis on mindfulness, gentle mobility, and internal body awareness makes yoga very beneficial for dealing with a variety of issues. *Here's an in-depth look at who can benefit from somatic movement and why:*

1. Seniors Seeking Increased Mobility and Independence

As we age, our bodies naturally alter, such as losing muscle mass, stiffening joints, and losing flexibility. These alterations might cause discomfort, limited mobility, and an increased risk of falling. Somatic movement is very good for elders since it allows them to:

- Improve Flexibility and Joint Health: Gentle, controlled movements enhance joint fluidity, which reduces stiffness and makes daily actions like bending, reaching, and walking easier.
- Improve Balance and Coordination: By focusing on body awareness, somatic activities improve coordination and balance, all of which are critical for minimizing falls, a common cause of injury in older persons.

- Relieve Chronic Pain: Many seniors suffer from chronic pain due to arthritis, back problems, or other illnesses. Somatic exercises serve to relieve tension and retrain the nervous system, resulting in long-term pain relief.
- Foster Independence: By enhancing mobility, strength, and confidence, elders can extend their independence and quality of life.

2. Individuals Living with Chronic Pain

Chronic pain, whether caused by fibromyalgia, arthritis, or injury, is frequently the result of repeated patterns of tension and restricted movement. Somatic movement treats these concerns through:

- Releasing Muscular Tension: Gentle, repetitive movements allow the body to "unlearn" pain-inducing behaviors, reducing muscle tightness and discomfort.
- Retraining the Nervous System: Somatic practices use neuroplasticity—the brain's ability to generate new pathways—to replace painful actions with painless alternatives.
- Providing a Safe Alternative: Unlike high-impact or severe exercises, somatic movements are mild and adaptive, making them perfect for people who are unable to exercise due to pain.

3. Individuals with High Stress or Anxiety Levels

Modern living is frequently accompanied by stress, worry, and physical indications of these situations, such as tight shoulders, shallow breathing, or stomach problems. Somatic movement can benefit by:

- Relaxation is promoted through conscious breathing techniques and calm, thoughtful movements, which stimulate the parasympathetic nervous system and reduce the body's stress reaction.
- Reconnecting Mind and Body: Stress and anxiety can result in a gap between how the body feels and how the mind perceives. Somatic activities help to bridge this gap by promoting calm and self-awareness.
- Releasing Stress-Related Tension: Over time, stress builds up in the body, causing chronic tension in places such as the neck, back, and jaw. Somatic activities serve to relieve stress "hotspots," restoring ease and comfort.

4. People Recovering from Injuries or Surgery

Following an accident or surgery, the body may develop compensatory movement patterns that produce discomfort or limit mobility. Somatic movement promotes rehabilitation through:

- Rebuilding Muscle Coordination: Gentle, attentive workouts can assist restore efficient movement patterns that have been disturbed by injury.
- Reducing Scar Tissue Tension: Somatic motions promote mild stretching and mobility, which can help alleviate the stiffness commonly associated with surgical recovery.
- Restoring Movement Confidence: Injury can cause fear of re-injury, resulting in hesitant or guarded movements. Somatic practices foster trust in the body by fostering pain-free, deliberate movement.

5. Athletes Seeking Improved Performance and Injury Prevention

Athletes frequently strain their bodies to the maximum, which causes muscle imbalances, stress, and an increased risk of injury. Including somatic movement in an athlete's regimen can:

- Improve Body Awareness: Understanding how the body moves and feels can assist athletes to improve their technique and avoid overcompensation of specific muscle groups.

- Improve Recovery: Somatic activities promote relaxation and tension relief, allowing athletes to recover faster after strenuous training or tournaments.
- Prevent Injury: Somatic techniques lessen the risk of overuse injuries by identifying and correcting imbalances or limited movements.

6. People with Neurological Conditions

Neurological diseases such as Parkinson's disease, multiple sclerosis, and stroke frequently impair coordination, balance, and motor function. Somatic movement can offer great assistance by:

- Somatic exercises promote neuroplasticity, or the brain's ability to adapt and build new neural pathways, which improves coordination and motor skills.
- Enhancing Mobility: Gentle, mindful movements help to maintain or recover the range of motion, counteracting the stiffness and spasticity that are frequent in these diseases.
- Promoting Relaxation: Stress and frustration are common symptoms of many neurological diseases.

Somatic activities promote a sense of peace and acceptance.

7. Individuals with Postural Issues or Sedentary Lifestyles

Prolonged sitting, poor posture, and repetitive actions frequently result in muscle imbalances, stiffness, and discomfort. Somatic movement contributes to:

- Realign the Body: Somatic exercises assist restore alignment and balance by increasing awareness of posture and habitual movement patterns.
- Release Sitting Tension: Gentle stretches and movements can help alleviate the consequences of extended sitting, such as tight hip flexors, rounded shoulders, and a stiff lower back.
- Encourage Active Sitting and Standing: Somatic approaches educate people on how to effectively activate muscles throughout daily tasks, which reduces strain and weariness.

8. Individuals Interested in Personal Development and Mindfulness

Somatic movement is more than just a physical activity; it is also an exploration of one's own identity. For people interested in personal development, it offers:

- Exploring how the body feels and moves leads to a stronger feeling of self-awareness and authenticity.
- Mindful Living: Somatic movement concepts such as presence, intention, and ease influence daily interactions and habits in addition to the practice itself.
- Emotional Release: Movement is intimately linked to emotion. Somatic techniques can often help people release suppressed emotions, resulting in a sense of liberation and calm.

9. Professionals with High-Stress Jobs

Doctors, teachers, caregivers, and other professionals in demanding positions frequently experience burnout, physical stress, and emotional tiredness. Somatic movement can benefit them:

- Simple somatic exercises performed during breaks help relieve tension in areas such as the neck, back, and shoulders.
- Reduce Burnout Symptoms: Somatics' thoughtful and relaxing nature helps to offset the mental and emotional toll of high-pressure work.
- Restore Energy: Gentle movements energize the body without depleting it, providing a long-term refresh.

10. Individuals New to Exercise or with Limited Mobility

Somatic movement provides a friendly entrance point for persons who are new to fitness or have physical limitations.

- Accessibility: Most somatic exercises can be modified to accommodate various fitness levels and performed seated or lying down.
- Somatic activities promote confidence by focusing on what feels pleasant rather than reaching a specific objective.
- Encouraging Exploration: Somatic movement allows people to test their abilities without fear of rejection or failure.

Somatic movement is a transformative technique that addresses a variety of needs, including chronic pain relief, sports performance enhancement, stress management, and emotional well-being. Its versatility and emphasis on internal awareness make it available and beneficial to almost anyone, regardless of age, physical condition, or life circumstances. Individuals can benefit from incorporating somatic practices into their daily lives by feeling more at ease, vibrant, and connected to themselves.

CHAPTER 2: THE SCIENCE BEHIND SOMATIC MOVEMENT

How Somatic Workouts Influence The Neurological System

While the advantages of these exercises are frequently connected with physical outcomes such as increased flexibility, strength, and mobility, the impact of somatic practices on the nervous system is equally deep and critical to their efficacy. Understanding how somatic exercises affect the neurological system might help people, especially seniors, comprehend the tremendous mind-body connection that they promote.

The nervous system is the body's communication network, transferring messages between the brain, spinal cord, and other organs. It is divided into two primary parts: the central nervous system (CNS), which contains the brain and spinal cord, and the peripheral nervous system (PNS), which contains all other nerves that branch out to the limbs, organs, and tissues. The nervous system directs and regulates all bodily functions, from basic survival tasks like heartbeat and breathing to more complicated activities like movement, cognition, and emotion.

The nervous system has two main branches that affect the body's response to stress and relaxation:

- The sympathetic nervous system (SNS) The sympathetic nervous system, sometimes known as the "fight or flight" system, prepares the body for action in reaction to perceived dangers by increasing heart rate, blood pressure, and muscle tension.
- The parasympathetic nervous system (PNS) In contrast, the PNS is known as the "rest and digest" system, which promotes relaxation, slows the heart rate, and allows the body to recuperate and repair.

Somatic exercises attempt to regulate the nervous system by minimizing SNS overactivity and encouraging PNS restorative actions.

The Function of Somatic Exercises in Nerve System Regulation

Somatic activities, which involve gentle, mindful movements, breathing techniques, and focused body awareness, affect both the CNS and the PNS in distinct ways. Individuals who deliberately engage in slow, focused movements and pay great attention to physiological sensations generate a feedback loop that soothes the nervous system and promotes healthy neuronal responses.

1. Increasing Body Awareness (Proprioception)

One of the primary ideas of somatic exercises is to improve body awareness, also known as proprioception, which is the ability to perceive and understand one's own position in space. This awareness is essential for movement coordination and injury prevention, as well as nervous system modulation.

Somatic exercises increase people's awareness of their posture, breathing, and muscular tension, providing signals to the brain that assist reprogram the body's reaction to stress and movement. This improved proprioception aids in the retraining of the nervous system by encouraging better control of muscle activity and coordination. Somatic activities, such as mild stretches or regulated movements, stimulate the CNS to focus on sensory data from muscles and joints, allowing the body to move more freely and comfortably.

In seniors, increased awareness can enhance motor control and reduce the probability of falls or mishaps. It also helps to stimulate neuronal pathways that may have been dormant as a result of aging or physical inactivity, encouraging the nervous system to respond in a healthier manner.

2. Increasing Neuroplasticity

Neuroplasticity refers to the brain's ability to restructure itself by creating new neural connections. As people age, their brain's plasticity declines, making it more difficult to recover from accidents, manage pain, and adapt to new motions or changes in physical health. However, somatic exercises have been found to boost neuroplasticity by engaging the body in unique ways, allowing the brain to establish new pathways.

In the context of somatic activities, neuroplasticity is especially useful for changing movement patterns and alleviating chronic pain. For example, if a person has bad posture or inefficient movement patterns as a result of a previous injury or long-term suffering, somatic exercises can help the brain "relearn" healthier movement patterns, reducing pain and enhancing overall mobility.

Somatic techniques also activate the brain's emotional centers since they frequently involve connecting with the body's sensations and emotions. This connection can help lessen anxiety, fear, and stress, which can all lead to muscle tightness and pain. Individuals can enhance their ability to manage pain and stress by retraining the brain through mindful movement, which benefits both their mental and physical health.

3. Decreased Stress and Anxiety

Chronic stress contributes significantly to nervous system dysfunction. Prolonged activation of the SNS, which can occur as a result of stress, causes several physical and emotional health problems, including muscle tension, an accelerated heart rate, high blood pressure, and mental tiredness. Somatic activities serve to counteract the effects of stress by stimulating the parasympathetic nervous system (PNS).

Somatic techniques, which include slow, deliberate movements, aware breathing, and mindfulness, help to activate the parasympathetic nervous system. This promotes a sense of calm and relaxation by lowering heart rate, blood pressure, and muscle tension. This is especially crucial for seniors, as prolonged stress can worsen illnesses such as hypertension, heart disease, and chronic pain.

Breathing exercises, which are frequently included in somatic practices, have an important role in soothing the nervous system. Deep, diaphragmatic breathing stimulates the vagus nerve, a crucial component in the PNS. This sort of breathing encourages the body's natural relaxation response, which helps to reduce stress, increase sleep quality, and improve overall mood.

4. Pain Relief with Somatic Movement

Somatic exercises can also alleviate pain by relaxing the nervous system and assisting the brain in reinterpreting pain signals. Chronic pain in the body is often caused by the nervous system becoming "stuck" in a loop of heightened sensitivity. This could be caused by an injury, inflammation, or emotional stress. Somatic activities help the body's natural healing process by urging the brain to change its emphasis from pain to ease and comfort.

Exercises like mild stretching or moderate, controlled motions, for example, help relieve tension in the muscles and joints while the brain concentrates on non-pain sensations. Over time, this can retrain the brain to be less sensitive to pain. Furthermore, these exercises improve proper posture and alignment, which can help with chronic pain caused by poor movement habits or muscle imbalances.

5. Improving Balance and Coordination

The nervous system is directly responsible for maintaining balance and coordination. Somatic activities, which focus on slow, controlled motions, can help the brain absorb sensory information related to balance. Individuals who practice mindful movement increase the link between their brain and muscles, which can improve coordination and lessen the chance of falling, a significant issue among seniors.

Movements that use proprioception and focus on short, controlled movements assist the nervous system in activating the proper muscles for balance, lowering the risk of instability and injury.

Somatic exercises are not only good for increasing physical flexibility and strength, but they also have a significant impact on the nervous system. These exercises increase neuroplasticity, regulate the autonomic nervous system, reduce stress, relieve pain, and enhance balance and coordination by including mindful movement, breathwork, and body awareness. Somatic techniques can improve elders' quality of life by increasing movement, lowering discomfort, and promoting emotional and mental well-being. Seniors who incorporate somatic exercises into their daily routine can maximize the potential of their nervous system, allowing them to live more active, pain-free, and balanced lifestyles.

The Connection Between The Body And Mind

The connection between the body and the mind is one of the most significant features of human existence. This connection, also known as the mind-body link, is essential for how we perceive, experience, and respond to our surroundings. It affects our physical health, emotional well-being, and overall quality of life. Modern science, ancient philosophies, and various therapeutic techniques have all dug into this complex relationship, revealing its significance and providing tools to harness its potential for healing and personal development.

The body-mind connection is fundamentally the interaction between our mental states (thoughts, emotions, and attitudes) and our bodily health and functioning. It expresses the idea that what we think and feel can directly affect our physiological state, and vice versa. Stress, as an emotional or psychological response, can cause physical symptoms such as headaches, muscle tightness, and even long-term diseases like hypertension. Similarly, physical conditions like chronic pain or disease can have an impact on mental health, potentially leading to anxiety or despair.

The neurological, endocrine, and immunological systems all play a role in mediating this link. These systems communicate bidirectionally, forming a dynamic feedback loop that keeps the body and mind in constant dialogue.

The body-mind link is not just a philosophical idea; it is supported by a wealth of empirical evidence.

1. Stress Response and Health: When the brain detects a threat, it initiates the "fight or flight" response via the hypothalamic-pituitary-adrenal (HPA) axis. This causes the release of stress chemicals such as cortisol and adrenaline, which prime the body for action.
1. Chronic activation of this reaction owing to chronic stress can have a deleterious influence on physical health, resulting in illnesses such as cardiovascular disease, impaired immunological function, and metabolic disorders.

2. The Role of Neurotransmitters: Neurotransmitters such as serotonin and dopamine play important roles in both mental and physical health. For example, low serotonin levels are linked to depression and anxiety, but they also have an impact on gut health because the majority of serotonin is produced in the gastrointestinal tract.

3. The Placebo Effect: The placebo effect is a striking example of the body-mind link. When people believe

they are getting effective treatment, their symptoms usually improve—even if the treatment is ineffective. This phenomenon demonstrates the impact of attitudes and beliefs on physical health.

4. Psychoneuroimmunology
5. This branch of study focuses on how psychological conditions affect the immune system. According to research, stress and negative emotions can impair immunological function, but good emotions and mindfulness techniques can improve it.

6. The Gut-brain Axis: The gut-brain axis is a two-way communication mechanism between the central nervous system (brain and spinal cord) and the enteric nervous system (gut). It emphasizes how gut health affects mood and cognition, and vice versa. This link is so strong that the gut is commonly referred to as the "second brain."

Emotions serve as an important link between the body and the mind. They develop from our interpretations of internal and external stimuli and manifest themselves both intellectually and physically. For example:

- Fear may cause a quick heartbeat and stiff muscles.

- Sadness might seem like exhaustion or a heavy feeling in the chest.
- Joy frequently causes an accelerated heart rate and a feeling of lightness.

These physical expressions of emotions demonstrate how inextricably linked our mental and physical states are. Suppressing emotions can result in unresolved stress in the body, which may contribute to persistent discomfort or sickness. In contrast, noticing and processing emotions can help to promote healing and reduce stress.

Mindfulness techniques like meditation, yoga, and tai chi are effective methods for improving the body-mind connection. These techniques emphasize being present at the moment and encouraging people to pay attention to their thoughts, feelings, and body sensations without judgment. According to research, mindfulness can

- Reduce stress and anxiety.
- Enhance attention and emotional regulation.
- Reduces blood pressure and heart rate.
- Improve immunological function.

Mindfulness also encourages interoception, or the ability to detect and comprehend internal body feelings such as hunger, thirst, and discomfort. Improved interoception can lead to greater self-care and stress management.

Somatic practices, such as somatic exercises, somatic experiencing, and other body-awareness therapies, aim to reconnect people with their bodies. These methods acknowledge that trauma, stress, and bad emotions can get "stuck" in the body, causing physical and emotional pain.

Somatic techniques urge people to release tension, improve posture, and restore body-mind harmony through gentle, mindful movements and body scans. These activities can be especially beneficial to elders in terms of chronic pain management, mobility improvement, and anxiety reduction.

Stress is a major disruptor of the body-mind relationship. Prolonged stress can have a variety of harmful bodily repercussions, including inflammation, hormone imbalances, and reduced immunity. Conversely, lowering stress can help to restore equilibrium and enhance general health. Techniques like this:

- Deep breathing activates the parasympathetic nervous system, which promotes relaxation.
- Progressive Muscle Relaxation: Lowers physical stress.
- Cognitive-Behavioral Therapy (CBT): Treats negative thought patterns that cause stress.

These methods show how regulating emotional states can improve physical health.

Here are some practical ways to strengthen the body-mind connection:

1. Exercise produces endorphins, which improve mood and alleviate pain. Yoga and tai chi integrate movement and attention, strengthening the body-mind connection.

2. Journaling: Writing down your ideas and feelings might help you digest them and clear your mind.

3. Healthy Nutrition: A well-balanced diet benefits both physical health and mental clarity. Foods high in omega-3s, for example, are known to improve brain function.

4. Sleep Hygiene: Adequate sleep is essential for preserving the body-mind link. Sleep allows the brain to process emotions while the body repairs itself.

5. Therapeutic Practices: Therapies such as somatic experiencing, acupuncture, and massage can help you relax and release accumulated stress.

While the body and mind are naturally intertwined, the following circumstances might disturb this relationship:

- Chronic stress overwhelms the neurological system, making it difficult to maintain balance.
- Trauma can cause a detachment from physical sensations as a coping technique.
- Sedentary behaviors, poor diet, and digital distractions all contribute to a weaker body-mind connection.

Recognizing and overcoming these problems is critical to restoring peace. The interaction between the body and mind is powerful and dynamic, influencing all parts of our lives. Understanding and fostering this link can benefit our physical health, emotional resiliency, and general sense of well-being. Whether via mindfulness, somatic practices, or simply paying attention to how we move and feel, developing the body-mind connection allows us to live healthier, more balanced lives. This relationship has the potential to be transformative for elders, assisting them in managing pain, reducing stress, and regaining a sense of vitality and purpose.

Neuroplasticity's Impact On Pain Relief And Movement

Neuroplasticity, also known as brain plasticity, is the brain and nervous system's amazing ability to restructure itself through the formation of new synaptic connections. This plasticity enables the brain to change its shape and function in response to new information, experiences, and injuries. Neuroplasticity plays an important part in the brain's ability to regulate chronic pain and improve motor performance. The brain's ability to remodel and adjust for injury or dysfunction is critical to rehabilitative therapies, particularly for people with chronic pain issues or motor impairments.

Neuroplasticity refers to the brain's ability to modify its structure in response to inputs, experiences, or external circumstances. It includes the development of new synapses (neuronal connections) as well as the strengthening or weakening of existing ones. Neuroplasticity occurs throughout life, although the brain's potential to reorganize itself is strongest during childhood. However, studies have revealed that adults can also experience major changes in brain structure and function.

There are two types of neuroplasticity: functional plasticity and structural plasticity.

- Functional plasticity refers to the brain's ability to transfer functions from damaged to undamaged regions.
- Structural plasticity refers to physical changes to the brain's structure caused by learning or experience, such as the production of new synapses or the growth of new neurons.

Neuroplasticity is necessary for adaptive learning, memory, and recovery from injury. It assists the brain in adjusting to new events and situations, and it is also an important aspect of trauma rehabilitation, including physical traumas or neurological impairment.

Neuroplasticity in the Setting of Chronic Pain

Chronic pain, defined as discomfort lasting longer than three months, can be a crippling condition that reduces an individual's quality of life. It is frequently caused by injury, inflammation, or chronic health issues. However, the brain's feeling of pain is not solely a result of tissue injury. Repeated pain signals can cause neuroplastic changes in the brain that affect how it interprets pain, even after the underlying lesion has healed.

Central sensitization is a key factor in persistent pain. Central sensitization occurs when the central nervous system (CNS) becomes overly sensitive to stimuli. Essentially, the brain becomes more sensitive to pain signals, increasing pain perception even in the absence of continuous tissue injury. This means that the brain may begin to perceive non-painful stimuli, such as touch or pressure, as painful.

Neuroplasticity underpins central sensitization, as the brain's neural connections are "rewired" to increase pain sensitivity. This maladaptive plasticity can lead to a vicious cycle in which pain repeats itself. However, the same plasticity that causes chronic pain also provides an avenue for treatment.

Neuroplasticity and Pain Relief

The good news is that neuroplasticity can function in reverse. The brain's plasticity also enables the "reprogramming" of neuronal circuits, which can diminish pain perception. Rehabilitative therapies that use neuroplasticity aim to teach the brain to perceive pain differently, lessen sensitivity, and improve movement.

1. Pain-Reprocessing Therapy: Pain reprocessing therapy is a developing topic in pain management that makes use of the concept of neuroplasticity. This technique focuses on assisting people in retraining their brains to perceive pain signals in new ways. Pain reprocessing, which employs approaches such as cognitive behavioral therapy (CBT), mindfulness, and graded exposure to movement, seeks to retrain the brain to lessen chronic pain through beneficial neuroplastic changes.

2. Motor Imagery and Movement Re-education: Neuroplasticity also plays an important role in motor rehabilitation following an injury. Motor imagery and workouts that engage the brain in specific movement patterns have been found to enhance neural plasticity. For example, simply picturing a movement, such as flexing a finger or moving an arm, can engage the same brain networks as actual physical movement. This means that rehearsing movement using mental imagery or modest physical exercises can help re-establish motor pathways, making movement smoother and less painful in the long run.

3. Graded Exposure to Movement: Gradual exposure to movement, beginning with modest, painless movements, aids in the re-engagement of the brain's

motor circuits. As the individual improves, the brain "learns" that movement does not always equal pain, potentially breaking the cycle of chronic pain. These steady, controlled movements are intended to generate neuroplastic changes that make movements smoother and less painful.

4. Mind/Body Therapies: Somatic activities, yoga, and Tai Chi are examples of mind-body methods that rely on the neuroplasticity concept. These practices combine physical activity with mindfulness to increase awareness of the body and the present moment. Gentle exercise not only improves physical flexibility and strength but also allows the brain to build new neural connections, which improves pain management and movement control.

Neuroplasticity in Movement

Neuroplasticity is important not just for pain alleviation, but also for increasing motor performance, especially following neurological traumas or age-related decrease. When a person has a stroke, a spinal cord injury, or another neurological illness, portions of the brain that control motor function may be destroyed. However, the brain may compensate for the injury by restructuring neuronal networks. Neurorehabilitation is a procedure in which people can retrain their brains to execute lost motions.

1. Rehabilitation Following Injury: Following neurological traumas such as a stroke, the brain can "remap" motor control. For example, if a section of the motor cortex that controls hand movement is damaged, another portion of the brain may take up that role. Targeted workouts and therapies can help the brain establish new pathways to restore motor function. Neuroplasticity allows the brain to regain lost talents, even years after an injury.

2. Repetitive, Task-Specific Training: One of the most effective methods to use neuroplasticity for mobility rehabilitation is through repetitive, task-specific training. The more frequently a person executes a specific activity, the more likely the brain is to create or strengthen neural connections that support it. For example, teaching a person to walk again after a stroke may entail repetitious exercises that focus on the exact activities required for walking. This repetitive practice gradually improves motor pathways, resulting in better movement and coordination.

3. Sensory Feedback and Motor Control: To direct motor control, the brain uses sensory data (such as proprioception or body position). Neuroplasticity enables the brain to adapt to changes in sensory information and modify movement accordingly. Patients suffering from peripheral neuropathy (nerve damage resulting in a lack of sensation in the feet or hands) might, for example, employ proprioceptive training to regain a sense of body position and motor control.

Neuroplasticity is an effective tool for pain alleviation and movement rehabilitation. The brain's ability to restructure and generate new neural connections provides hope to those suffering from chronic pain or motor limitations. Neuroplasticity can be harnessed through focused therapies, exercises, and mindful practices to relieve pain, restore movement, and improve overall quality of life. Seniors, in particular, can preserve mobility, regain function, and live pain-free lives by engaging in somatic exercises and other neuroplasticity-based therapy on a consistent basis.

CHAPTER 3: SAFETY FIRST

Creating A Safe And Pleasant Atmosphere For Practice

Somatic exercises focus on creating a deep connection between the mind and body through gentle, focused movement. For seniors over the age of 60, having a safe and comfortable atmosphere is critical to allowing them to completely benefit from these activities without risk of injury or discomfort. A well-prepared practice area ensures not only physical safety but also mental calm, which is essential for the efficiency of somatic workouts. Below, we'll look at the fundamental components of creating such an environment.

1. Choosing the Right Space

The first step in creating a secure and comfortable workplace is to choose a suitable site for your practice. The space should match the following criteria:

a. Quiet and Calm Environment: Find an area free of distractions, noise, and interruptions. A calm setting improves focus and helps seniors connect to their bodies' sensations. If feasible, select a space with soft lighting or natural light to create a relaxing atmosphere.

b. Enough Space for Movement: Make sure there is adequate space to move around without knocking against furniture or other obstructions. It is advised to leave at least 6-8 feet of clean space surrounding the practice area. If you're exercising with a chair or a mat, be sure they're stable and secure.

c. Accessibility: The room should be easily accessible to elders, particularly those who have mobility issues. Avoid staircases and areas with uneven flooring. For wheelchair users, make sure the space is wide enough to accommodate the chair and any additional equipment.

2. Setting up the Surface

The workout surface is critical to safety and comfort. Consider the following aspects when preparing the practice area:

a. Non-slip Flooring: A non-slip mat or yoga mat can be used to cushion and prevent slippage during sitting or laying movements. Avoid practicing on smooth or slippery surfaces, such as tiles or glossy wood, without a suitable mat.

b. Stable Chair Support: For workouts that require sitting, choose a solid chair with a flat seat and no wheels. Chairs with armrests can offer extra assistance if necessary. To keep the chair from moving while in use, place it on a sturdy, non-slip surface.

c. Cushioned Support: If reclining exercises are included, make sure the mat or floor is adequately cushioned to avoid discomfort, especially for seniors with sensitive joints or back concerns. Use additional cushions or bolsters to provide support in certain areas, such as under the knees or in the lower back.

3. Creating a Relaxing Environment

A comfortable atmosphere promotes relaxation and the mind-body connection. Consider the following elements to create a relaxing practicing environment:

a. Temperature Control: Maintain a moderate room temperature to avoid feeling cold or overheating when exercising. Provide blankets or warm clothes for elders who may become chilly during the relaxation or cooling periods.

b. Lighting: Choose gentle, diffused lighting to create a peaceful mood. Natural light is preferred, but if it is not accessible, use warm-toned bulbs instead of harsh fluorescent lighting. Avoid using very bright or glaring lights, which may cause discomfort or distraction.

c. Sound and Music: Gentle background music or nature sounds can help you relax and focus. To avoid distractions, use tunes that do not have lyrics. Alternatively, some elders may prefer silence to focus solely on their motions and breathing.

d. Aromatherapy: Relaxation can be promoted by using lightly scented candles or essential oil diffusers with calming fragrances such as lavender or chamomile. Ensure that the odors are not overbearing and are suitable for people with sensitivities.

4. Setting Up for Accessibility

Accessibility is critical for ensuring that seniors of all physical capacities can participate in somatic activities safely and comfortably.

a. Changing the Environment: For seniors with restricted mobility, provide chairs with enough support and make sure activities may be adapted to a seated posture if necessary. Place any necessary equipment, such as water bottles, props, or music remote controls, in easy reach.

b. Supportive Assistance: If possible, have a family member, caregiver, or teacher available to aid, especially if you need help transitioning between positions or staying balanced.

c. Visual and Auditory Aids: Ensure that instructions for seniors with hearing or vision impairments are clear and simple to understand. Visual clues and simple hand motions can be useful. Avoid cluttered environments with excessive patterns or bright colors, as these can be unsettling for people with visual impairments.

5. Promoting Mental Comfort

A safe and comfortable atmosphere not only ensures physical safety but also promotes mental and emotional calm. Here's how to establish a supportive mental environment:

a. Positive Reinforcement: Encourage senior citizens to listen to their bodies and develop self-compassion. Remind them that somatic activities are about gentle exploration, not perfectionism. Provide confidence that they can change or cease motions as needed.

b. Mindfulness Practices: To set a tranquil tone for the session, start with a moment of mindfulness or deep breathing. Encourage individuals to pay attention to their bodily feelings and move at their own pace.

c. Eliminating Pressure: Avoid time limits and highly regimented routines, which can induce stress. Emphasize the significance of enjoying the process.

6. Testing and Adjusting the Space

Once the room is set up, it is crucial to test it out and make any necessary adjustments:

a. Trial Practice: Perform a few basic activities to confirm that the room fulfills all safety and comfort standards. Pay attention to any discomfort or impediments that may develop while moving.

b. Feedback: If you're an instructor or caregiver, solicit comments from the senior practicing in the space. Their feedback might assist improve the arrangement for maximum comfort.

c. Regular Maintenance: Periodically inspect the area for wear and tear on equipment or matting to ensure everything is in excellent working order.

To have a pleasant and effective practice, seniors over the age of 60 must create a safe and comfortable setting for somatic exercises. By emphasizing safety, accessibility, and relaxation, you can ensure that each session promotes physical well-being and emotional peace. A well-prepared environment not only reduces the chance of harm but also improves the overall experience, allowing seniors to reconnect with their bodies and receive the full advantages of somatic movement.

Basic Safety Recommendations To Avoid Injury

Somatic workouts can be revolutionary for elders, providing pain alleviation, stress reduction, and increased mobility. However, like with any physical exercise, safety must come first to avoid injuries. Somatic exercises are low-impact by nature, but appropriate technique and creating the ideal environment are critical for a safe and effective session. Here, we look at basic safety measures to assist seniors do somatic workouts safely and confidently.

1. Know Your Body's Limits

The foundation of somatic training is listening to and respecting your body's limitations. Seniors sometimes contend with illnesses such as arthritis, osteoporosis, or chronic pain, which can limit their movements. Pushing the body beyond its capacity can result in injuries like muscular strains or joint pain.

How To Practice Safely:

1. Start with simple exercises to determine your body's readiness and flexibility.
2. Pay attention to pain signals. Pain is the body's way of communicating pain. If an activity causes pain or discomfort, stop immediately and alter the movement.

3. Somatic workouts emphasize adaptation. Modify exercises to fit your range of motion and comfort level.

2. Create a Safe and Comfortable Environment

The environment in which you do somatic exercises is critical in preventing accidents. Seniors must exercise in a safe environment to avoid the chance of falls or injury.

Tips for Safe Setup:

1. Remove any impediments, such as carpets, cords, or furniture, that could cause tripping.
2. Choose non-slip surfaces. To ensure stability during exercises, use a yoga mat or nonslip flooring.
3. Make sure the area is well-lit to limit the possibility of mistakes.
4. If you are concerned about your balance, practice near a sturdy chair or wall for extra support.

3. Wear the Proper Attire

What you wear during somatic workouts can affect your safety. Restrictive clothing or improper footwear can limit movement and cause accidents.

Recommendations:

1. Wear loose-fitting, breathable clothing that allows for complete range of motion.
2. Many somatic exercises are performed barefoot or with nonslip socks to increase grounding and stability. If going barefoot is uncomfortable, wear nonslip socks.
3. For standing exercises, use shoes with arch support and nonskid soles.

4. Warm Up Before Starting

Warming up is an important phase that many people ignore, yet it prepares the body for exercise and helps to avoid injuries. A decent warm-up boosts blood flow to muscles, relaxes joints, and improves flexibility.

Effective Warm-Up Techniques:

1. Use gentle stretches to target key muscle groups such as the neck, shoulders, and back.
2. Deep, regular breathing exercises can help oxygenate the body and soothe the nervous system.
3. Simple exercises like shoulder rolls or seated marches can gently stimulate muscles and joints.

5. Use Props and Equipment Correctly

To increase comfort and support, somatic workouts may include props like chairs, resistance bands, or yoga blocks. Using these tools incorrectly can result in strain or falls.

Guidelines for Safe Prop Use:

1. If workouts require a chair, be sure it's stable and doesn't wobble. Avoid using wheeled chairs unless they are properly fastened.
2. To avoid snapping, use bands with adequate resistance levels and inspect for tears.
3. Use cushions or yoga blocks to provide additional support and alignment while sitting or lying down.

6. Maintain Appropriate Posture and Alignment

Incorrect posture during somatic activities can put undue strain on joints and muscles, increasing the likelihood of injury. Maintaining adequate alignment ensures that movements are both effective and safe.

Tips for Good Posture:

1. Maintain a natural, relaxed posture with no undue arching or rounding.
2. Lightly contract the abdominal muscles to help support the lower back and maintain stability.
3. Avoid clenching your shoulders, jaw, or fists while exercising.

7. Pace Yourself

Somatic workouts are supposed to be slow and thoughtful, allowing the body to gradually adjust to new motions. Rushing through workouts might damage form and cause accidents.

How to Pace Yourself:

1. Use deep, steady breaths to control the pace of your motions.
2. Pause between workouts to assess how your body is feeling and avoid overexertion.
3. Begin with easier exercises and work your way up to more difficult moves as you gain confidence.

8. Stay Hydrated

Staying hydrated is critical for preserving muscle flexibility and avoiding cramps, particularly for seniors who are more susceptible to dehydration.

Tips for Hydration:

1. Drink water 15-30 minutes before exercise.
2. Keep a water bottle nearby to stay hydrated during your workout.
3. Drinking modest amounts of water will help you prevent feeling bloated or heavy.

9. Be Aware of Pre-existing Conditions

Many seniors have chronic health concerns like arthritis, sciatica, or high blood pressure, which might limit their ability to undertake specific workouts. Before beginning any new workout routine, consult with a healthcare professional.

What to consider:

1. Get medical clearance before exercising, especially if you've recently had an injury or surgery.

2. Work with a somatic instructor to customize movements to meet your individual needs.
3. Be mindful of how medications may impair your balance, energy levels, or coordination.

10. Monitor Your Breath and Heart Rate

Paying attention to your breathing and heart rate can help you prevent overexertion and stay calm and focused throughout somatic workouts.

To improve breathing awareness, avoid holding your breath. To avoid unneeded tension, breathe naturally and consistently.
Sync Movement with Breath: Use inhalations and exhalations to control the flow of your movements.

Monitor heart rate and maintain a comfortable pace. Avoid exhausting yourself.
Pause if needed. If you feel dizzy or weary, stop and rest.

11. Cool Down After Your Workout

Cooling down is equally vital as warming up. It helps the body shift from exercise to relaxation, minimizing muscle soreness and preventing stiffness.

Cooling Down Tips:

1. Do mild stretches to relieve tension in the muscles engaged throughout your workout.
2. Try somatic relaxation techniques like lying flat and focusing on calm, deep breathing.
3. Drink plenty of water and allow yourself to rest before returning to your normal routines.

12. Seek Advice When Needed

While somatic workouts are simple to learn, a teacher can help you do them safely and successfully.

Benefits of Professional Guidance:

1. An instructor can detect incorrect motions and make changes.
2. Classes or tutorials offer a defined framework to follow.
3. Professional support can help beginners gain confidence.

Safety is of the utmost importance when performing somatic workouts, particularly for elders. Understanding your body, maintaining a safe setting, and using the right techniques allow you to reap the full advantages of these workouts while reducing your chance of injury. Remember that the purpose of somatic workouts is not only to improve physical mobility but also to promote relaxation and well-being. Approach each movement attentively, listen to your body, and enjoy the road to better health and balance.

Proper Warm-Up Techniques To Prepare The Body

A proper warm-up is a crucial part of any exercise routine, especially for seniors who participate in somatic workouts. Warming up gets the body ready for exercise by gradually increasing circulation, enhancing flexibility, and activating muscles. Warm-up activities are especially important for seniors over the age of 60 since they help prevent injuries, relieve stiffness, and improve mobility. A well-structured warm-up also prepares the mind, resulting in a focused, calm condition required for the attentive motions of somatic exercises.

Warming up is more than just a preamble to a workout; it's an essential technique that prepares the body for safe and productive activity. *Here are several major advantages of warming up:*

1. Increases Blood Flow: Gentle movements during a warm-up improve blood circulation, ensuring that muscles receive enough oxygen and nutrients to perform properly.
2. Loosens Stiff Joints: Warm-ups lubricate joints, smoothing out movements and lowering the chance of strain or discomfort.

3. Activates the Neurological System: A correct warm-up alerts the neurological system to get ready for exercise, which improves coordination and response time.

4. Injury Prevention: Warm-ups reduce the risk of strains, sprains, and other injuries by gradually developing flexibility and mobility.

5. Improves Mental Focus: Practicing mindful warm-up exercises helps seniors connect with their bodies, allowing them to approach their workout with awareness and intention.

Components of an Effective Warm-up

An efficient warm-up should gradually prepare the entire body, with special emphasis on areas prone to stiffness or tension. Warm-ups for somatic workouts should focus on slow, deliberate movements that adhere to mindfulness and body awareness principles.

1. Gentle Cardiovascular Activity: Start with light motions to boost heart rate and circulation. This could include seated marching, arm swings, or slow strolling on the spot.

2. Dynamic Stretches: Use continuous, controlled motion to loosen joints and muscles. Examples include shoulder

rolls, modest side-to-side neck movements, and hip circles.

3. Mindful Breathing: Combine movement with deep, diaphragmatic breathing to boost oxygen levels and reduce stress. This encourages relaxation while ensuring that the muscles are properly prepared.

4. Joint Mobilization: Perform movements to mobilize joints, such as wrist rotations, ankle circles, and moderate knee bends. These activities are especially beneficial for elders suffering from stiffness or arthritis.

5. Core Activation: Warming up the core muscles improves balance and stability. Simple exercises, such as seated pelvic tilts and mild spine rotations, can safely stimulate these muscles.

Example Warm-Up Routine for Somatic Workouts

The following is a step-by-step warm-up routine for seniors over 60. This practice takes 8-10 minutes and can be customized to meet individual needs.

1. Seated Marching (2 Minutes)

1. Sit in a solid chair, feet flat on the floor.
2. Simulate a marching motion by gently lifting one knee at a time.

3. Swing your arms lightly in time with your legs.
4. Keep your motions moderate and steady, and keep your posture upright.

The purpose of this workout is to enhance circulation, engage the legs, and warm up the arms.

2. Shoulder Rolls (1 Minute)

1. Sit or stand comfortably, arms relaxed at your sides.
2. Slowly move your shoulders forward in a circular motion 5-10 times.
3. Reverse the direction and roll your shoulders back.

Shoulder rolls assist relieve stress in the neck and shoulders while also increasing joint mobility.

3. Neck Mobility (One Minute)

1. Sit or stand erect, head in a neutral position.
2. Slowly tilt your head to one side, placing your ear near your shoulder. Hold for a breath, then return to the center.
3. Repeat on the opposite side.

4. Gently turn your head to gaze over your shoulder before returning to the center. Repeat on the other side.

These motions relax the neck and increase the range of motion, eliminating stiffness.

4. Spinal Warm-Up with Cat-Cow (1 Minute)

1. Sit on the edge of a chair, hands resting on your thighs.
2. Inhale as you arch your back slightly, elevate your chest, and look up (Cow Pose).
3. Exhale as you round your back and drop your chin into your chest (Cat Pose).
4. Repeat this exercise 5-8 times in synchrony with your breathing.

This moderate workout warms up the spine, increasing flexibility and decreasing stress.

5. Hip Circles (1 Minute)

1. Sit or stand, hands on hips for support.
2. Slowly move your hips in small circles clockwise for 5-10 times.
3. Reverse the direction and repeat.

The purpose of hip circles is to release the hips and pelvis, which are necessary for mobility and balance.

6. Ankle and Wrist Rolls (1 Minute)

1. Sit comfortably and raise one foot off the ground.
2. Gently spin your ankle in a circular motion 5-10 times, then reverse direction.
3. Repeat for the opposite ankle.
4. For the wrists, stretch your arms in front of you and rotate them in both directions.

These motions improve circulation and mobility in the extremities, hence reducing stiffness.

7. Seated Side Stretch (1 Minute)

1. Sit tall on your chair, feet level on the ground.
2. Place one hand on the edge of the chair for support while raising the opposite arm overhead.
3. Lean gently toward the supporting side, experiencing a stretch across your body.
4. Hold for 2-3 breaths, then repeat on the opposite side.

The purpose of this stretch is to warm up the sides of the torso and increase spinal flexibility.

Tips for Safe and Effective Warm-Ups

1. Begin Slowly: Always start with mild movements to avoid overstressing cold muscles. Gradually increase the intensity as your body warms up.
2. Listen to Your Body: Take note of how your body feels during the warm-up. Stop or change any movement that produces discomfort or suffering.
3. Maintain Consistency: Regardless of how light or tough your workout is, a full warm-up should always be included in your regimen.
4. Practice Mindfulness: Focus your mind on the sensations in your body and the rhythm of your breathing.
5. Hydrate: Make sure you're properly hydrated before beginning your warm-up, as dehydration can impair muscle performance and flexibility.

Common Mistakes to Avoid During Warm-Ups

1. Skipping the Warm-Up: Starting exercise without properly preparing your body raises the chance of injury and diminishes workout efficiency.

2. Rushing Through Movements: Warm-ups must be slow and deliberate in order to be successful. Rushing is counterproductive to the goal of preparing the body.
3. Overstretching Cold Muscles: Stretching too deeply at first can strain the muscles. Concentrate on energetic, delicate motions instead.

A thorough warm-up is a necessary component of any somatic activity, particularly for seniors. It not only prepares the body for exercise, but it also improves mental focus and decreases the likelihood of damage. Seniors can make their workouts safer, more successful, and fun by integrating moderate, mindful activities like seated marching, shoulder rolls, and spinal stretches. Prioritizing a warm-up ritual promotes a stronger connection between the body and mind, laying the groundwork for long-term health and well-being.

CHAPTER 4: BREATHING TECHNIQUES FOR CALM AND RELAXATION

Breathing is one of the most basic activities of life, but it is sometimes disregarded as a potent tool for improving mental and physical health. Learning to use effective breathing methods can help seniors reduce stress, relax, and improve their overall health. These strategies are especially beneficial when combined with somatic exercises since they strengthen the link between the body and mind.

Breathing is directly related to the autonomic nerve system, which regulates involuntary body activities like heart rate, digestion, and stress reaction. This system is divided into two branches: the sympathetic nervous system (which controls the "fight or flight" reaction) and the parasympathetic nervous system (which controls the "rest and digest" response). When we are stressed, our sympathetic nervous system becomes active, resulting in quick, shallow breathing, elevated heart rate, and enhanced awareness.

In contrast, deep and focused breathing activates the parasympathetic nervous system, causing the body to relax. This response reduces stress chemicals like cortisol, lowers blood pressure, and slows the heartbeat. Engaging the parasympathetic system through breathing can be life-changing for seniors who are already stressed by health issues, limited mobility, or social isolation.

In addition, breathing has a direct impact on the brain. Deep, regular breathing boosts oxygen flow to the brain, improving mental clarity and emotional equilibrium. It stimulates the vagus nerve, which connects the brainstem to the abdomen, promoting relaxation and lowering anxiety.

Advantages of Proper Breathing Techniques for Seniors

1. Decreased Stress and Anxiety: Mindful breathing relaxes the nervous system and helps seniors deal with daily challenges. They may control their emotional responses to difficult events by focusing on breathing.

2. Enhanced Sleep Quality: Many seniors suffer from insomnia or restless sleep. Relaxation-focused breathing before bedtime can help you get a better night's sleep by relieving mental and physical strain.

3. Improved Mobility and Pain Relief: Deep breathing relaxes stiff muscles, boosts oxygen delivery, and improves circulation, all of which can help relieve joint and muscular pain. This is especially effective when combined with somatic motions.

4. Improved posture and lung capacity: Conscious breathing helps good posture by encouraging spinal alignment and chest openness. It can gradually increase lung function and capacity, hence boosting overall respiratory health.

5. Improved Emotional Resilience: Learning to focus on the breath gives elders a sense of control, allowing them to better deal with feelings of impatience, fear, or despair.

Practical Breathing Techniques for Calm and Relaxation

Here are some breathing techniques that promote relaxation and serenity. They can be done in any calm area, as a stand-alone activity, or as part of a somatic fitness regimen.

1. Diaphragmatic (Belly) Breathing

How to Practice:

1. Sit or lie comfortably.
2. Put one hand on your chest, and the other on your abdomen.
3. Inhale deeply via your nose, expanding your abdomen rather than your chest. The hand on your abdomen should rise while the hand on your chest stays static.
4. Slowly exhale through your lips, gently squeezing your abdominal muscles to expel the air.
5. Repeat for 5–10 minutes.

Benefits: This technique improves oxygen flow, decreases tension, and promotes deep relaxation.

2. Box Breathing (Four Square Breathing)

How to Practice:

1. Sit up straight in your chair or lie down in a relaxed position.
2. Inhale through your nose four times.
3. Hold your breath for four counts.
4. Exhale through your mouth four times.
5. Hold your breath for four counts before restarting the cycle.

6. Continue for 5 minutes.

Benefits: Box breathing helps quiet the mind, improve attention, and prepare for sleep.

3. Alternate nostril breathing (Nadi Shodhana)

How to Practice:

1. Sit comfortably and close your eyes.
2. Put your thumb over your right nostril and breathe strongly through your left nose.
3. Close your left nostril with your ring finger, then remove your thumb from the right nostril and exhale via the right nostril.
4. Inhale through the right nostril and then exhale through the left.
5. Repeat for 3–5 minutes.

Benefits: This practice reduces anxiety, clears the mind, and promotes balance.

4. The 4-7-8 Breathing Technique

How to Practice:

1. Find a comfortable sitting or lying position.
2. Inhale gently through your nose for a count of four.
3. Hold your breath for a count of seven.
4. Exhale strongly through your mouth for a count of eight.
5. Repeat for four cycles, progressively increasing as you feel comfortable.

Benefits: This approach relieves tension and lowers heart rate quickly.

5. Guided Visualization

How to Practice:

1. find a quiet location and sit or lie down comfortably.
2. Close your eyes and start breathing slowly and deeply.
3. Imagine a relaxing scene, such as a beach or a forest, with each inhalation delivering fresh air and each exhale relieving tension.
4. Concentrate on the subtleties of the sight, such as the sound of waves, the rustle of leaves, or the warmth of the sun.

5. Continue for ten minutes.

Benefits: This approach promotes inner peace by calming the mind and reducing unpleasant emotions.

Integrating Breathing Techniques into Daily Life

Breathing exercises work best when done consistently. Here are some suggestions for incorporating them into a senior's everyday routine.

- Morning Routine: Start your day with a 5-minute diaphragmatic breathing session to establish a calm and concentrated tone.
- During stressful situations, practice box breathing or alternating nostril breathing to instantly relieve tension and regain attention.
- Pre-Exercise: Use breathing techniques to warm up the body and mind before engaging in somatic motions.
- Before bed, use 4-7-8 breathing or guided visualization to relax and encourage healthy sleep.

Breathing is an effective yet simple strategy for encouraging calm and relaxation, especially for seniors dealing with the physical and mental challenges of aging. Seniors who practice techniques such as diaphragmatic breathing, box breathing, and alternate nostril breathing can improve their overall well-being, handle stress, and connect more deeply with their bodies. These exercises not only supplement somatic training but also provide a road to a more tranquil and balanced lifestyle.

CHAPTER 5: THE POWER OF SLOW, CONTROLLED MOVEMENT

How To Move With Intention And Awareness

Movement is an essential part of our daily lives, but many of us go through the motions without really engaging or being aware of our actions. When we walk, stretch, or complete a task, we frequently do it on autopilot, which can lead to inefficiency, discomfort, and even damage over time. Moving with intention and awareness is a discipline that can change the way we interact with our bodies and the environment around us. It is a fundamental idea in somatic exercises, yoga, Pilates, and other mindful movement activities that center on drawing attention to the body and the sensations it feels while moving.

Intention in movement means having a clear and deliberate direction for the activity you are performing. This is determining what you want to achieve with that movement, whether it's flexibility, strength, pain treatment, or simply engaging in the current moment. Intention entails bringing mindfulness to the activity itself, being clear about your goal for each motion, and coordinating your physical efforts with your mental and emotional focus.

Awareness, on the other hand, means being present in the moment while you move. This includes paying attention to how your body feels, how the muscles and joints react, and any sensations, whether good or unpleasant. It's about paying attention to your body and observing its signals, rather than becoming distracted or alienated from what's going on physically.

When we mix intention and awareness in our movements, we develop a stronger connection to our bodies. This exercise can help us move more efficiently, avoid injuries, and develop a sense of peace.

The following are the benefits of moving with intention and awareness:

1. Increased Body Awareness: One of the key benefits of moving with intention is that it makes you more aware of how your body moves in space. When you practice mindful movement, you become more aware of your posture, alignment, and muscle activation, which can aid in correcting imbalances or bad movement patterns.

2. Improved Efficiency: Intentional movement is frequently more efficient than unthinking, mindless motion. When you

focus on your body's alignment, breathing, and muscle engagement, you may discover that things become easier and less exhausting since you use less energy to complete them. This can result in increased stamina and a feeling of lightness in the body.

3. Pain Relief and Injury Prevention: Many injuries result from unconscious, repetitive actions that strain-specific muscles or joints. Moving with awareness can help you detect areas of stress or misalignment in your body, allowing you to make adjustments and avoid harm. Somatic exercises, in particular, highlight awareness as a significant role in pain management by teaching people how to move in ways that reduce tension and increase mobility.

4. Stress Reduction: Intentional movement promotes mindfulness, which has been linked to reduced stress and anxiety. When you are in the present moment and focused on how your body feels, you are less likely to become obsessed with external pressures. This can help you relax and feel calm.

5. Better Posture and Alignment: By paying attention to how you hold and move your body, you can gradually improve your posture and alignment. This is especially useful for

elders or anyone who is in pain due to bad posture or muscular imbalances.

To walk with intention and awareness, examine these guiding principles:

1. Start with Breathing

Before you start any physical activity, you should concentrate on your breathing. Breathing is the foundation of conscious movement, connecting the mind and body. Inhale deeply through your nose, filling your lungs with air, then exhale completely via your mouth or nose. This relaxes the nervous system and tells your body that it's time to be present and intentional. To retain a sense of flow and connection while moving, strive to match your breathing with your movements.

Tip: Breathe diaphragmatically, expanding your abdomen as you inhale and softly contracting it as you exhale. This form of deep breathing can help to relieve stress and promote relaxation.

2. Focus on the Quality of Movement

Rather than hurrying through exercises or chores, focus on the quality of each movement. Ask yourself: *How do my muscles feel as I move? Are my joints appropriately aligned? Is there tension or strain in any portion of my body?* Slow down and pay attention to the sensations of each movement, aiming for smoothness, fluidity, and control.

Tip: When stretching, for example, halt at the place when you feel a little stretch and hold that position. Take a few breaths in this position and watch how your muscles lengthen and relax.

3. Cultivate Mindful Posture

Your posture is the basis for all movement. Proper body alignment can help to prevent strain and discomfort. To practice mindful posture, begin by assessing your alignment before moving. For example, stand with your feet hip-width apart, shoulders relaxed, and head in line with your spine. Imagine a string pushing the top of your head toward the ceiling, generating a sense of length and space throughout your spine.

Tip: If you notice yourself drooping or rounding your shoulders, gently return your awareness to an aligned posture while keeping your spine straight and your chest wide.

4. Move Slowly and with Purpose

Moving with intention often entails slowing down. Rushing through motions can lead to a loss of awareness and contribute to muscle tightness or bad posture. Instead, attempt to move slowly, especially when stretching, doing strength exercises, or walking. Slower movements allow you to assess how your body is behaving and modify accordingly.

Tip: Slowly perform movements like squats and lunges, holding each position for a few seconds to deepen muscle engagement and develop alignment awareness.

5. Pay Attention to the Sensations in Your Body

As you move, pay close attention to how your body feels. *Is there tension? Is one side of your body stiffer than the other? Are you holding your breath?* Take note of any discomfort or ease as you move between positions. This awareness enables you to make modifications, such as easing into a stretch or shifting your body to avoid tension.

Tip: If you experience pain or discomfort while exercising, pause and check your position. Adjust your movement such that it is both comfortable and effective, without forcing it.

6. Use Visualization Techniques

Visualization is a strong tool for moving with intention. Before starting an activity, imagine how you want your body to move. Consider the muscles you want to use, the joints you need to maintain, and the area you need to fill with energy. This mental preparation helps you focus on the work at hand and generates a clearer path for your body to take.

Tip: Before doing a sitting leg raise, imagine your leg moving easily and without tension, concentrating on activating the muscles in your thigh and core.

7. Reflect and Adjust

After completing a movement or workout, take time to consider how it feels. *Were there any places of tension or discomfort that could be alleviated with increased awareness? Were there any actions that felt especially effortless or natural?* This thought enables you to improve your technique over time, making each action more deliberate and effective.

Tip: Keep a notebook to record how different exercises or movements make you feel, and then alter your practice accordingly.

Moving with intention and awareness is a transforming activity that improves the quality of your physical motions while also improving your mental clarity and emotional well-being. Slowing down, breathing intentionally, and tuning into your body can help you connect more deeply with yourself and the world around you. This conscious approach to movement results in increased efficiency, pain relief, improved posture, and reduced stress. Whether you're doing a somatic workout, stretching, or simply strolling, applying intention and awareness to each action can help you move more easily, confidently, and calmly.

Understanding The Significance Of Pacing

Pacing is an important notion in somatic exercises, especially for seniors, because it directly affects the effectiveness, safety, and overall enjoyment of a workout. Pacing is vital for somatic exercises since they focus on awareness, bodily connection, and moderate movement, preventing excessive strain on the body. Pacing is especially important for seniors because it considers age-related changes in mobility, muscle strength, flexibility, and overall health.

Pacing relates to the rate, intensity, and duration with which a person performs physical activities or exercises. Pacing in somatic exercises is the intentional management of movement rate to fit the body's current physical state, allowing for safe, successful, and joyful practice. This includes being aware of not only how rapidly one moves, but also how long a specific movement lasts and how much effort is put into each motion. Proper pacing allows the body to perform exercises without overstretching, overexerting, or putting excessive strain on the muscles or joints.

Pacing for seniors is more than just slowing down exercises to avoid injury; it also includes time for muscular activation, relaxation, and recovery, all of which are essential components of somatic practices. It encourages thorough listening to the body, indicating when it's time to slow down or when it's ready for a little more activity.

Why Pacing is Important for Seniors

Muscle mass, joint health, flexibility, and endurance all naturally vary as people get older. Pacing becomes critical for staying comfortable, enhancing mobility, and preventing overuse injuries. *Here's why elders need to pace themselves:*

1. Prevents Injury: The most obvious advantage of pace is that it prevents injuries. As we age, our tissues become less resilient, increasing the risk of muscular strain or joint overstretching. Seniors can avoid putting too much stress on sensitive muscles and ligaments by timing their movements carefully and gently. This helps to prevent overexertion and strain, both of which can cause pain or even long-term harm.

2. Improves Movement Quality: Somatic exercises focus on quality rather than quantity. When elders move slowly and deliberately, they gain a better understanding of how their bodies accomplish each activity. This allows them to make minor tweaks that can significantly increase the efficiency and alignment of their movement. Proper pacing promotes a stronger

connection with the body's senses, which improves posture, joint alignment, and general movement patterns. By focusing on quality, elders can gradually retrain their bodies to move more effectively, lowering discomfort and increasing usefulness.

3. Supports Muscle Activation and Relaxation: A common error elders make when beginning an exercise routine is racing through the movements to finish it fast. However, haste can keep the muscles from fully activating or releasing. Somatic exercises focus on muscle engagement and release. Pacing permits these processes to go effectively. When elders pace themselves, they allow their muscles to progressively activate, ensuring that they are using the proper muscles and not compensating with other portions of the body. Similarly, pacing ensures that muscles have enough time to fully relax, reducing tension and increasing flexibility.

4. Improves Flexibility and Mobility: Flexibility and mobility naturally deteriorate with aging. Slow, deliberate movement, on the other hand, aids in the recovery and maintenance of these abilities in elders. Seniors who pace somatic activities allow their bodies to gently stretch and release tension without forcing movement.

Slow movements allow the joints to loosen up, resulting in improved range of motion and flexibility over time. This controlled pace is more successful at improving mobility because it encourages safe and steady progress, which reduces the risk of strain or damage.

5. Promotes Relaxation and Stress Relief: One of the primary advantages of somatic exercises is their capacity to alleviate stress and anxiety. When elders take the time to pace their movements and breathe deeply, they can activate the parasympathetic nerve system, which controls the body's rest-and-digest response. Moving slowly and deliberately allows elders to attain a state of mindfulness that promotes relaxation. The pacing slows the heart rate, lowers blood pressure, and produces a sense of peace, which is especially good for seniors who are anxious or stressed.

6. Encourages the Mind-Body Connection: Somatic activities are based on body awareness and mindfulness. When seniors practice activities carefully, they can become more aware of how their muscles feel, where tension is stored, and how their joints move. This increased awareness can lead to better self-care practices and help seniors detect areas that require further attention, such as discomfort, tightness, or

stiffness. Pacing fosters a mind-body connection, allowing seniors to make more educated judgments about how much effort to exert and when to rest.

7. Avoids Overexertion: Overexertion is a prevalent problem for many seniors who try to push themselves too hard during exercise, especially when they follow the pace of a younger or more physically fit individual. This can cause weariness, pain, and even damage. Pacing is vital when performing somatic exercises to prevent elders from overworking their bodies. Slower movements help them to stay within their physical boundaries, avoiding pushing too hard or too quickly. This allows elders to exercise safely, knowing when to ease up and when to push a little harder within their limits.

How to Pace Somatic Exercise Effectively

Pacing effectively in somatic exercises involves practice, patience, and self-awareness. *Here are some useful strategies to assist seniors to pace their movements:*

1. Begin Slowly and Build Gradually: Start with basic, gentle movements. Avoid speeding through exercises, particularly in the early stages. Begin with a few minutes

of stretching or light movement, then gradually increase the duration as you feel more comfortable.

2. Concentrate on Breathing: Pacing relies heavily on breathing. Deep, controlled breathing helps regulate the body's tempo and promotes relaxation. Focus on thoroughly exhaling, allowing the body to relax and slow down.

3. Listen to Your Body: Pay attention to any soreness or weariness symptoms. If a movement is too difficult, slow down, take a break, or adjust it. Avoid pushing yourself past your boundaries.

4. Incorporate Rest Periods: Allow plenty of rest between workouts to allow the muscles to heal. Somatic exercises are intended to be restorative, and regular rests allow the body to digest the motions without overworking the muscles.

5. Use Time as a Measure: Instead of racing through sets or repetitions, take the time to pace yourself. Set a timer for a specified amount of time for each exercise or movement, and concentrate on the quality of the movement during that period.

Pacing is more than just moving slowly; it's about moving wisely and deliberately. Pacing allows seniors who practice somatic exercises to connect with their bodies on a deeper level, lowering the chance of injury, increasing flexibility, and improving general health and well-being. Seniors can get the benefits of somatic exercises by taking the time to pace their movements properly, respecting their physical limits, supporting healing, and promoting long-term health. Finally, pacing results in a more enjoyable, lasting, and effective exercise experience.

CHAPTER 6: GENTLE HEAD AND NECK SOMATIC EXERCISES

1. Neck Rolls

Instructions:

1. Sit or stand up straight with your shoulders relaxed and your head aligned with your spine.
2. Gently lower your chin toward your chest.
3. Slowly roll your head in a circular motion, first to the left, and then around to the back, right, and finally back to the starting position.
4. After completing one rotation, reverse the direction by rolling your head to the right.
5. Perform 5 to 10 rolls in each direction, making sure to keep the movement slow and fluid, avoiding any jerks.

2. Shoulder Shrugs

Instructions:

1. Stand or sit with your back straight and arms relaxed at your sides.
2. Slowly lift your shoulders toward your ears as if trying to touch them with your ears.
3. Hold the position for a second, then gently release and lower your shoulders back to the starting position.
4. Repeat the movement for 10 to 15 repetitions, making sure to focus on a smooth, controlled motion.
5. To intensify, you can hold light weights in your hands while performing the shrugs.

3. Neck Stretch

Instructions:

1. Sit upright with your back straight and shoulders relaxed.
2. Gently tilt your head to the right, bringing your ear toward your shoulder.
3. Hold this stretch for 15-30 seconds, feeling a mild stretch on the left side of your neck.
4. Slowly return to the center and repeat on the left side.
5. Perform 2-3 sets on each side to improve flexibility.

4. Shoulder Circles

Instructions:

1. Stand or sit with your back straight and arms extended at your sides.
2. Slowly make small circles with your shoulders, moving them forward.
3. Gradually increase the size of the circles, then reverse the direction and make circles backward.
4. Perform 10-15 circles in each direction.
5. Keep your core engaged and maintain smooth, controlled movements throughout the exercise.

5. Seated Levator Scapula Stretch

Instructions:

1. Sit on a chair with your feet flat on the ground and back straight.
2. Place your left hand on the base of your head, and gently tilt your right ear toward your right shoulder.
3. Using your left hand, gently apply pressure to the back of your head to deepen the stretch.

4. Hold for 20-30 seconds, feeling a stretch along the left side of your neck and upper back.
5. Switch sides and repeat the stretch for another 20-30 seconds.

6. Shoulder Hunch and Release

Instructions:

1. Sit or stand with a straight posture and arms relaxed at your sides.
2. Gently roll your shoulders forward, bringing them up toward your ears in a hunching motion.
3. Hold the hunch for a second, then relax and release your shoulders downward, opening your chest.
4. Repeat this movement 10-15 times, focusing on engaging the shoulder muscles throughout.
5. Ensure each release is slow and controlled to maximize the stretch and relieve tension.

7. Supine Spinal Extension

Instructions:

1. Lie on your back with your arms extended overhead and legs straight.
2. Inhale deeply, and as you exhale, gently lift your chest off the floor and extend your arms toward the ceiling.
3. Keep your lower back pressed into the floor as you extend your spine, creating a gentle curve from the base of your spine upward.
4. Hold the extended position for 5-10 seconds, then slowly return to the starting position.
5. Perform 8-12 repetitions to gently stretch and relax the spine.

8. Neck Isometrics

Instructions:

1. Sit upright with your shoulders relaxed.
2. Place your left hand against the left side of your head, just above the ear.
3. Push your head into your hand, resisting the motion with your hand for 5-10 seconds.
4. Relax briefly, then repeat the process, switching sides.

5. Perform the exercise 3-5 times on each side to strengthen neck muscles.

9. Trunk-Shoulder Differentiation

Instructions:

1. Sit or stand with a straight back and relaxed shoulders.
2. Keeping your shoulders relaxed, gently rotate your upper trunk to the left without moving your lower body.
3. Hold the position for a moment, then return to the center.
4. Repeat the motion on the right side.
5. Perform this exercise 10-15 times on each side, ensuring that only the torso rotates while the lower body remains still.

CHAPTER 7: GENTLE BACK SOMATIC ACTIVITIES

---

10. Back Lift

Instructions:

1. Lie flat on your back with your knees bent and feet flat on the floor, hip-width apart.
2. Place your arms at your sides, palms facing down.
3. Press your feet into the floor, engage your glutes, and lift your hips toward the ceiling, creating a straight line from your knees to your shoulders.
4. Hold the lifted position for a few seconds, then gently lower your hips back to the floor.
5. Repeat for 8-12 repetitions, ensuring the movement is controlled and steady.

11. Somatic Side Bend Variation

Instructions:

1. Sit comfortably with your spine straight and legs extended or crossed.
2. Place your left hand on the floor beside you, and raise your right arm overhead.
3. Slowly lean your torso to the left, feeling a gentle stretch along the right side of your body.
4. Hold the position for 15-30 seconds, then slowly return to the starting position.
5. Repeat on the other side, alternating between both sides for 3-5 repetitions each.

12. Sphinx

Instructions:

1. Lie on your stomach with your forearms on the floor, elbows aligned directly under your shoulders.
2. Press into your forearms and gently lift your chest off the floor, arching your back and keeping your lower body relaxed.
3. Keep your head aligned with your spine, looking straight ahead, and hold the position for 20-30 seconds.

4. Breathe deeply, keeping your torso lifted and chest open.
5. Lower back down slowly and repeat for 3-5 repetitions, making sure to move gently.

13. Child's Pose with Reach

Instructions:

1. Start by kneeling on the floor with your knees apart and your big toes touching.
2. Lower your hips back toward your heels and stretch your arms forward on the floor.
3. As you reach forward, keep your forehead resting on the floor for a deeper stretch.
4. Hold for 20-30 seconds, then slowly return to a kneeling position.
5. Repeat 2-3 times, feeling the stretch along your back, arms, and shoulders.

14. Lower Back Pain Reliever

Instructions:

1. Lie on your back with your knees bent and feet flat on the floor.
2. Gently hug your knees into your chest while keeping your lower back on the floor.
3. Slowly rock your body back and forth in a gentle motion to massage your lower back.
4. Hold the position for 10-15 seconds, then slowly release and repeat 3-5 times.
5. If comfortable, add small circles with your knees to increase the relief.

15. The Boomerang

Instructions:

1. Sit with your legs extended straight in front of you and your spine straight.
2. Bend your knees slightly and place your hands behind you for support.
3. Lift your hips off the floor, then slowly move your legs forward and backward in a controlled, swinging motion.

4. Focus on smooth and controlled movement, ensuring the spine remains long and straight.
5. Perform 8-10 repetitions for gentle movement, then rest.

16. Inversion/Eversion

Instructions:

1. Sit with your legs straight in front of you and feet flexed.
2. Slowly turn your feet outward (eversion) by bringing the soles of your feet toward the floor.
3. Reverse the motion by pointing your feet inward (inversion), bringing the soles together.
4. Perform 10-15 slow and controlled repetitions in each direction.
5. Keep your legs relaxed while isolating the movement to your feet and ankles.

17. Superman Pose

Instructions:

1. Lie face down on the floor with your arms extended overhead and legs straight.
2. Engage your core and slowly lift your arms, chest, and legs off the floor, keeping them straight and extended.

3. Hold for 3-5 seconds, squeezing your lower back and glutes as you lift.
4. Slowly lower back to the floor, ensuring smooth, controlled movement.
5. Repeat for 8-10 repetitions, focusing on the engagement of your back and core muscles.

18. Twisted Curl

Instructions:

1. Sit on the floor with your knees bent and feet flat.
2. Place your hands behind your head and engage your core.
3. Slowly rotate your torso to the left, bringing your right elbow toward your left knee.
4. Return to the center and repeat on the other side, bringing your left elbow toward your right knee.
5. Continue alternating sides for 10-15 repetitions, maintaining slow, controlled movements.

CHAPTER 8: MILD SOMATIC EXERCISES FOR THE ARMS AND CHEST

19. Chest Opener

Instructions:

1. Stand or sit with your spine straight and shoulders relaxed.
2. Interlace your fingers behind your back and straighten your arms, palms facing inward.
3. Slowly lift your arms away from your body, gently opening your chest, and squeeze your shoulder blades together.
4. Hold the stretch for 15-30 seconds, breathing deeply to enhance the stretch.
5. Slowly release and repeat for 2-3 sets.

20. Wall Angels

Instructions:

1. Stand with your back against a wall, feet about 6 inches away from the base.
2. Press your lower back, upper back, and head against the wall while keeping your knees slightly bent.
3. Bring your arms to a 90-degree angle, with elbows bent and the backs of your hands touching the wall.
4. Slowly slide your arms upward, keeping the backs of your hands and arms in contact with the wall.
5. Lower your arms back to the starting position and repeat for 10-15 repetitions.

21. Chest Expansion

Instructions:

1. Stand with your feet hip-width apart, and interlace your fingers behind your back.
2. Straighten your arms and gently lift them away from your body, opening your chest and stretching your shoulders.
3. Lift your chest upward as you press your palms together, pulling your shoulder blades down and back.

4. Hold for 15-30 seconds, breathing deeply to maximize the stretch.
5. Slowly release and repeat for 2-3 sets.

22. Spinal Arch and Flatten

Instructions:

1. Sit on a chair with your feet flat on the floor and hands resting on your knees.
2. As you inhale, arch your back, tilting your pelvis forward and lifting your chest upward.
3. As you exhale, flatten your spine by pulling your belly button toward your spine and rounding your back slightly.
4. Continue the movement in a slow, controlled manner for 10-15 repetitions, syncing with your breath.
5. Focus on the smooth articulation of your spine and core engagement.

23. Seated Pectoral Muscles Stretch

Instructions:

1. Sit on a chair with your feet flat on the floor and your spine straight.
2. Place your hands behind your head and gently open your elbows out to the sides.
3. Slowly pull your elbows back to feel a stretch across your chest and shoulders.
4. Hold for 15-30 seconds, breathing deeply to release tension in the pectoral muscles.
5. Release and repeat 2-3 times, focusing on deepening the stretch with each exhale.

24. Butterfly Hug

Instructions:

1. Sit comfortably with your feet flat on the floor and your spine tall.
2. Place your hands on your shoulders with your elbows bent and facing outward.
3. Slowly bring your elbows forward toward each other, crossing them gently in front of your body.

4. Open your elbows wide, feeling a stretch across your chest and shoulders.
5. Repeat for 8-12 repetitions, focusing on slow and controlled movements.

25. Wrist Curls

Instructions:

1. Sit comfortably with your feet flat on the floor and a lightweight or resistance band in each hand.
2. Rest your forearms on your thighs or a table with your wrists hanging off the edge.
3. With your palms facing up, curl your wrists upward, lifting the weight or resistance band.
4. Slowly lower your wrists back down to the starting position.
5. Perform 10-15 repetitions for each hand, ensuring smooth and controlled movement.

26. Tricep Pandiculation

Instructions:

1. Sit or stand tall with your arms extended overhead.
2. Slowly bend your elbows and bring your hands down toward your shoulders, keeping your elbows stationary.

3. Press your hands gently into your shoulders, engaging your triceps as you resist the motion.
4. Hold for 5 seconds, then release.
5. Repeat for 8-10 repetitions, focusing on controlled movement and engagement.

27. Arm Flexion and Extension

Instructions:

1. Sit or stand with your feet flat on the floor and your arms extended in front of you at shoulder height.
2. Slowly bend your elbows to bring your hands toward your shoulders (flexion).
3. Then, extend your arms straight out again (extension), keeping your elbows locked.
4. Continue alternating between flexion and extension for 10-15 repetitions, maintaining smooth, controlled motions.
5. Keep your shoulders relaxed and focus on the movement from your elbows and forearms.

28. Bicep Pandiculation

Instructions:

1. Sit or stand with your arms extended in front of you at shoulder height.
2. Slowly bend your elbows, bringing your hands toward your shoulders, and tense the biceps.
3. Hold the contraction for 3-5 seconds, then release slowly.
4. Repeat for 8-10 repetitions, focusing on slow, controlled engagement and release.
5. Maintain a relaxed neck and shoulders throughout the movement.

CHAPTER 9: SOFT SOMATIC TECHNIQUES FOR THE PELVIC REGION AND ABDOMENS

---

29. Pelvic Tilt

Instructions:

1. Lie flat on your back with your knees bent and feet flat on the floor, hip-width apart.
2. Tighten your abdominal muscles and gently tilt your pelvis upward, flattening your lower back against the floor.
3. Hold the position for 5-10 seconds while breathing deeply, then relax.
4. Repeat 10-15 times, focusing on engaging your core and moving your pelvis slowly.
5. This movement can be modified by placing your hands on your lower abdomen to feel the muscles working.

30. Abdominal Breathing

Instructions:

1. Sit comfortably or lie on your back with your knees bent.
2. Place one hand on your chest and the other on your abdomen.
3. Slowly inhale through your nose, allowing your belly to rise as your diaphragm expands, without lifting your chest.
4. Exhale through your mouth, allowing your abdomen to fall and the air to leave your lungs completely.
5. Repeat for 5-10 minutes, focusing on slow, deep breaths and relaxing your body.

31. Psoas Release

Instructions:

1. Lie flat on your back with your knees bent and feet flat on the floor.
2. Place one hand on your lower abdomen, and the other on the top of your thigh or knee.
3. Gently press your thigh away from your body, feeling a stretch along the front of your hip.
4. Hold the stretch for 20-30 seconds, then relax and repeat 2-3 times on each side.

5. This stretch helps to release tension in the psoas muscle, which is essential for maintaining good posture and mobility.

32. Pelvic Clock

Instructions:

1. Lie on your back with your knees bent and feet flat on the floor.
2. Visualize a clock face on your abdomen, with your belly button in the center.
3. Slowly tilt your pelvis toward noon, then move it to 3 o'clock, 6 o'clock, and 9 o'clock in a circular motion.
4. Keep your back relaxed, and only move your pelvis to the limit of your comfort.
5. Perform the exercise for 5-10 minutes, switching directions halfway through.

33. Cat-Cow

Instructions:

1. Start on your hands and knees with your wrists directly beneath your shoulders and knees beneath your hips.
2. Inhale as you arch your back, lifting your head and tailbone toward the ceiling (Cow Pose).
3. Exhale as you round your back, tucking your chin toward your chest and your pelvis toward your belly button (Cat Pose).
4. Repeat for 10-15 cycles, moving slowly and synchronizing your breath with the movement.
5. Focus on articulating each vertebra, from your tailbone to your neck.

34. Supine Leg Lift

Instructions:

1. Lie flat on your back with your knees bent and feet flat on the floor.
2. Slowly extend one leg straight out while keeping your back pressed firmly against the floor.
3. Lift the extended leg 6-8 inches off the floor, engaging your core.

4. Hold for 5-10 seconds, then lower the leg slowly back to the floor.
5. Repeat for 10-15 repetitions on each leg, ensuring smooth, controlled movements.

35. Inward-Outward Legs

Instructions:

1. Lie on your back with your knees bent and feet flat on the floor.
2. Lift both legs off the floor, keeping your knees bent at a 90-degree angle.
3. Slowly move your legs outward away from each other, then gently bring them back together.
4. Repeat for 10-15 repetitions, focusing on controlled movement and engaging your core.
5. Keep your back flat on the floor to avoid any unnecessary strain.

36. Bridge Pose

Instructions:

1. Lie on your back with your knees bent and feet flat on the floor, hip-width apart.
2. Press through your heels and lift your hips toward the ceiling, keeping your shoulders and feet grounded.
3. Engage your glutes and thighs as you lift, and hold for 5-10 seconds.
4. Slowly lower your hips back to the floor and repeat for 10-15 repetitions.
5. To deepen the stretch, try holding the pose for longer periods and focusing on breathing deeply.

37. Long Leg Psoas Release

Instructions:

1. Lie on your back with one leg extended straight and the other knee bent.
2. Hold the knee of the bent leg to your chest, keeping the extended leg straight on the floor.
3. Gently press your lower back into the floor, feeling a stretch in the hip flexors and psoas muscle of the extended leg.
4. Hold the stretch for 20-30 seconds, then switch legs.

5. Perform this stretch for 2-3 sets on each leg to release tension in the hip flexors.

38. Supine Spinal Twist

Instructions:

1. Lie on your back with your arms extended out to the sides and knees bent.
2. Slowly drop both knees to one side while keeping your shoulders grounded on the floor.
3. Turn your head in the opposite direction, creating a gentle twist along your spine.
4. Hold for 20-30 seconds, then return to the center and switch sides.
5. Repeat for 2-3 sets, focusing on deep breathing and gentle stretching.

CHAPTER 10: GENTLE SOMATIC EXERCISES FOR THE FEET AND LEGS

39. Tibia Toe Raises

Instructions:

1. Stand tall with your feet hip-width apart, and knees slightly bent.
2. Slowly lift your toes towards the ceiling, keeping your heels on the ground.
3. Hold at the top for 1-2 seconds, then slowly lower your toes back down.
4. Repeat for 10-15 repetitions, focusing on controlled movement.
5. You can place your hands on a sturdy surface for balance if needed.

40. Thigh and Hamstring De-escalation

Instructions:

1. Sit on the floor with your legs extended straight in front of you.
2. Gently flex your feet and point your toes upwards.
3. Reach forward toward your toes with your arms, gently stretching your hamstrings.
4. Hold the stretch for 20-30 seconds, focusing on relaxing into the stretch.
5. Repeat 2-3 times, keeping your back straight and avoiding any jerking motions.

41. Side Bend

Instructions:

1. Stand tall with your feet hip-width apart and, arms at your sides.
2. Raise one arm overhead and gently lean to the opposite side, feeling the stretch along the side of your torso.
3. Hold the stretch for 20-30 seconds, breathing deeply to enhance the stretch.
4. Return to the starting position, and repeat on the other side.

5. Perform 3-5 repetitions on each side, moving slowly and gently.

42. Foot Pandiculation

Instructions:

1. Sit comfortably in a chair with your feet flat on the floor.
2. Stretch your legs out in front of you and point your toes as far as you can.
3. Then, flex your feet, pulling your toes toward your shins.
4. Hold each position for 5-10 seconds, alternating between flexing and pointing your toes.
5. Repeat for 10-15 cycles, paying attention to the feeling in your feet and lower legs.

43. Standing Forward Fold

Instructions:

1. Stand tall with your feet hip-width apart, and knees slightly bent.
2. Hinge at the hips, lowering your torso toward the floor, and keeping your spine straight.
3. Let your head and neck relax, and try to touch your toes or the floor with your hands.

4. Hold the position for 15-30 seconds, breathing deeply into the stretch.
5. Slowly return to standing by rolling up one vertebra at a time.

44. Washrag

Instructions:

1. Stand tall with your feet shoulder-width apart.
2. Extend your arms in front of you, keeping them straight.
3. Slowly twist your torso to the right, then to the left, as if wringing out a wet rag.
4. Focus on moving from your waist while keeping your hips stable.
5. Perform 10-15 repetitions on each side, keeping the movements controlled.

45. Seated Ankle Flexion

Instructions:

1. Sit in a chair with your feet flat on the floor and knees bent at 90 degrees.
2. Lift one foot off the floor and flex your ankle so that your toes point toward your shin.

3. Hold the position for 3-5 seconds, then slowly return to the neutral position.
4. Repeat 10-15 times on each foot, focusing on controlled movement.
5. For an added stretch, point your toes away from your body before flexing them back.

46. The Flower

Instructions:

1. Sit with your legs crossed in a comfortable position.
2. Place the soles of your feet together and gently press your knees toward the floor.
3. Hold your feet with both hands and slowly open your legs wider, resembling the petals of a flower.
4. Breathe deeply as you gently hold the stretch for 20-30 seconds.
5. Repeat 2-3 times, ensuring you don't force your knees too far down.

47. Iliotibial (IT) Band Relief

Instructions:

1. Sit on the floor with your legs extended straight in front of you.
2. Cross one leg over the other, placing your foot flat on the floor.
3. Gently twist your upper body toward the crossed leg, placing your opposite elbow on the outside of the knee.
4. Hold for 20-30 seconds, feeling the stretch along the outside of your hip and thigh.
5. Repeat 2-3 times on each side, ensuring to move slowly and without jerking.

48. Seated Knee Circles

Instructions:

1. Sit comfortably in a chair with your feet flat on the floor.
2. Lift one knee off the ground and gently rotate it in a circular motion, clockwise for 10-15 rotations.
3. Repeat the motion in the opposite direction for 10-15 rotations.
4. Switch to the other knee and repeat the process.

5. Focus on moving from the hip joint and keeping the movement smooth and controlled.

CHAPTER 11: BUILDING A DAILY ROUTINE FOR FLEXIBILITY AND CALM

Creating A Routine For Incorporating Somatic Exercises Into Daily Life

Somatic exercises are an effective way to increase flexibility, relieve pain, reduce tension, and restore a sense of peace and well-being. These exercises, which emphasize attentive, body-centered movements, can be especially effective for seniors over 60 who suffer from chronic pain, stiffness, and mobility concerns. One of the keys to making somatic exercises effective is to incorporate them into daily life so that the benefits last beyond the exercise session and become part of a routine that improves general health and quality of life.

Developing a consistent, pleasurable, and sustainable program for somatic workouts is critical for long-term effectiveness. In this article, we'll look at how to create a daily schedule that works for you and makes somatic exercises a regular part of your day.

1. Begin with a Clear Intention and Goal

Before beginning your practice, you should understand why you're doing somatic exercises and what you aim to achieve. Seniors' aims may include pain alleviation, more flexibility, decreased worry, increased mobility, or simply a sense of well-being. Setting a clear intention helps you stay focused, motivated, and committed to your long-term health goals.

When developing a regimen, ask yourself the following:

- What's my primary goal? (For example, lowering back discomfort, enhancing posture, and relieving stress.)
- How would I like to feel after each session? (Examples: more calm, less tense, invigorated)
- What kind of progress would I like to track? (For example, increased flexibility, less pain, and better sleep.)

Starting with clear aims allows you to tailor your daily somatic routine to your health demands and lifestyle.

2. Start Slowly and Set Realistic Expectations

When introducing somatic exercises into your everyday routine, it is critical to begin cautiously. If you're new to somatics or haven't been physically active in a while, don't jump into a rigorous routine. The beauty of somatic exercises is their slow, deliberate tempo, which promotes deep body awareness and delicate movement. Over time, your body will adapt to these workouts, allowing you to gradually increase the intensity and complexity of your motions.

A recommended method is to start with 10-15 minutes of somatic exercises every day. As your body adapts and you get more comfortable with the motions, you can progressively increase the length of your workouts to 30 minutes or more. Remember that somatic exercises should never be painful; instead, they should be comfortable and relaxing. If you feel any discomfort or strain, alter the movements or reduce the intensity.

3. Consistency is Key

Setting up a steady schedule is one of the most efficient strategies to include somatic workouts in your everyday life. This does not imply that every day must be the same, but setting up a regular time in your day for these activities might help them become habits.

To establish a constant routine:

- Set aside a definite period each day for your somatic practice. Many individuals believe that practicing first thing in the morning sets a good tone for the rest of the day. Others might choose a noon or evening ritual to help them unwind.
- Set a reminder or add it to your daily schedule. Treat it as if it were a mandatory meeting or appointment.
- Begin small to prevent overwhelming yourself. Begin with short, manageable sessions that you may easily schedule into your day. As you become more comfortable, increase the duration.

4. Listen to Your Body

Somatic exercises are all about connecting with your body and moving with purpose. One of the most crucial components of this exercise is learning to listen to your body's signals. Unlike more traditional types of exercise, which may focus on pushing through discomfort or achieving a specific goal, somatic exercises allow you to be present and adjust your movements based on how you feel.

Throughout Your Routine:

- Pay attention to how your body feels during each workout. Recognize any areas of stress, discomfort, or tightness, and use your movements to gently relieve them.
- Adjust your movements according to how you feel at the moment. If you feel a stretch is too difficult, back off and try a gentler variety. Somatic movement is not about pushing boundaries, but rather about becoming more aware of your body's current state.
- Use your breath as a guideline. Deep, attentive breathing allows you to relax into the exercises while also guiding the pace and intensity of each movement. Breathe deeply and gently, paying attention to any tense or stressful parts of your body.

5. Mix It Up: Create Variety

While consistency is vital, variety in your routine is also essential for keeping things fresh and avoiding monotony. Somatic exercises can target different sections of the body, and changing up the activities you practice each day might help you avoid overstressing specific areas. It also helps you to alleviate any discomfort or tension that may emerge.

You can tailor your practice to target different sections of the body on different days. For example:

- Day 1: Gentle motions such as neck rolls, shoulder shrugs, and chest openers can help to strengthen the neck, shoulders, and upper back.
- Day 2: Stretch out your legs, tilt your pelvis, and release your hamstrings.
- Day 3: Include exercises that work the core and abdominal muscles, such as bridge postures and psoas releases.

Alternatively, you might combine movements for several regions of the body in a single session to avoid overworking any one muscle group.

6. Set Realistic Time Goals

As you begin to incorporate somatic exercises into your daily routine, it is critical to set realistic time targets. Begin by committing to a specific amount of time per day—whether it's 10, 15, or 20 minutes—and gradually increase the duration as you feel comfortable. The idea is not to finish as many exercises as possible, but to fully engage with each one, allowing your body to relax and restore.

If 15 minutes feels too long, consider breaking up your exercise into small periods. For example, you could do 5-minute morning and evening sessions with new exercises each time. This not only makes it easy to schedule time for somatic practice in your daily life, but it also helps you maintain consistency.

7. Track Your Progress

Tracking your progress helps you stay motivated and observe the results of your somatic practice. Keeping a simple notebook in which you describe how you feel before and after each session might provide useful information about how somatic exercises affect your body and mind.

In your journal, consider noting:

- Before the treatment, identify any areas of tension or pain.
- The type of activity you performed and how your body responded.
- Any increases in flexibility, movement, or relaxation.
- Emotional changes, such as reduced anxiety or stress levels.

Tracking success in this manner reinforces the benefits of your practice and encourages you to keep continuing.

Integrating somatic exercises into your daily routine can be quite beneficial for seniors, particularly in terms of pain alleviation, stress reduction, and increased mobility. Somatic exercises can become a regular part of your routine by starting slowly, listening to your body, making realistic goals, and staying persistent, thereby enhancing both your physical and emotional health. Whether you practice for 10 or 30 minutes a day, these gentle, mindful movements can help restore flexibility, tranquility, and well-being, resulting in a more pleasant, vibrant existence.

The Role Of Consistency In Restoring Mobility And Well-Being

Consistency is a tremendous force when it comes to gaining long-term mobility and overall well-being, particularly for seniors who participate in somatic exercises. While a single session may bring immediate alleviation or relaxation, it is the cumulative effect of consistent practice that results in deep and long-lasting changes.

1. Building Muscle Memory for Better Mobility

The human body thrives on repetition. Consistent somatic exercises serve to establish and maintain muscle memory, making motions more fluid and natural over time. This is especially crucial for the elderly, who may face stiffness, balance difficulties, or limited range of motion as a result of aging or inactivity.

With repeated practice, the brain and nervous system learn to optimize movement patterns, resulting in more efficient and effortless action. Gentle stretching and controlled movement exercises, for example, can help the body retrain itself to release chronic tension and regain lost flexibility. Over time, seniors may discover that previously difficult tasks, such as bending, reaching, or standing up, become easier and less painful.

2. Enhanced Neuroplasticity for Long-Term Pain Relief

One of the most intriguing elements of somatic workouts is their effect on neuroplasticity, the brain's ability to rearrange and generate new neural connections. Consistent practice enables the nervous system to "unlearn" maladaptive habits that cause pain or discomfort and replace them with healthier, more efficient ones.

For example, persistent pain is frequently associated with the brain misinterpreting signals from the body as a result of prolonged tension or bad posture. Regular somatic activity breaks the loop by educating the brain to notice and rectify negative tendencies. Over time, this lessens pain and increases total body awareness, resulting in a greater sensation of ease in everyday motions.

3. Gradual Increase in Flexibility and Range of Motion

Flexibility is not something that can be developed immediately; it requires patience and consistent practice. Consistent somatic practice softly stretches and lengthens muscles, allowing for an increased range of motion without tension. Unlike high-intensity workouts, which can lead to injuries, somatic exercises emphasize steady improvement, making them excellent for seniors with joint problems or mobility limitations.

For example, a senior who frequently performs pelvic tilts or modest spinal twists will see an improvement in their capacity to bend, turn, and rotate their body. These little but important advantages accumulate over time, making daily tasks like dressing, cooking, and gardening more fun and less physically demanding.

4. Strengthening the Mind-Body Connection

Somatic exercise is built on the mind-body connection, which is a conscious knowledge of how the body feels and moves. This connection strengthens with continuous practice, allowing seniors to better comprehend their body's signals and respond properly.

For example, frequent somatic exercises may assist seniors in identifying when they are retaining unneeded stress in their shoulders or clenching their jaw. By becoming more aware of these tendencies, they can deliberately relax in particular places, lowering stress and avoiding long-term discomfort.

Furthermore, a strong mind-body link promotes a feeling of empowerment. Seniors frequently report feeling more in charge of their physical health and well-being, which can be highly inspiring and empowering.

5. Increased Stability and Balance

Falls are a major worry for seniors, often resulting in injuries and a decrease in general mobility. Consistent somatic practice can dramatically minimize the likelihood of falling by improving balance, stability, and coordination.

Exercises that target core strength, alignment, and weight distribution help seniors maintain a more stable posture and respond more efficiently to rapid changes in position. Simple movements, such as shifting weight from one foot to the other, can help improve proprioception or the body's sense of position in space. This leads to improved control and fewer mishaps in everyday life over time.

6. Emotional and Mental Resilience

The benefits of consistent somatic practice go beyond physical wellness. Regular activity has a significant impact on mental and emotional health. Somatic activities help to relieve stress by activating the parasympathetic nervous system, which regulates rest.

Over time, regular activation results in a more balanced emotional state, making it simpler to handle anxiety, despair, or feelings of overwhelm. Furthermore, the contemplative nature of somatic exercises, which emphasize breathing and movement, promotes awareness, which can increase mental clarity and general life happiness.

7. Motivation Through Visible Progress

One of the most enjoyable benefits of sticking to a steady regimen is the ability to see and feel tangible results. Seniors frequently see improvements in their posture, energy levels, and pain management after just a few weeks of consistent exercise. These modest triumphs are huge motivators to keep going.

For example, a senior who initially fails to complete a sitting spinal twist may discover that with repeated effort, they can accomplish the action with increasing ease and range. This sensation of accomplishment creates a positive feedback loop, motivating even more commitment to their somatic practice.

8. Long-term Prevention of Age-related Decline

Aging is a normal process, but frequent somatic exercise can help delay or even reverse some of the effects. Seniors who engage in mild, restorative activities on a regular basis can retain their mobility, independence, and quality of life long into their later years.

Regular practice helps to combat the muscle stiffness, joint pain, and postural abnormalities that are common with age. Furthermore, it promotes cardiovascular health and circulation, ensuring that the body is well-supplied and capable of repairing itself.

9. Setting Up a Routine for Holistic Wellness

Consistency gives structure and regularity, which are necessary for overall well-being. Setting aside time for somatic practice regularly might help seniors feel more purposeful and stable in their everyday lives.

Whether it's a morning ritual to energize the body or an evening practice to unwind, incorporating somatic exercises into your daily routine guarantees that the benefits build up over time. This sense of predictability can also help to minimize stress and uncertainty, which improves general emotional well-being.

10. Social and Community Benefits

Consistency can help seniors who attend group somatic sessions or online communities form social connections. Sharing your progress, experiences, and encouragement with others fosters a sense of community and support.

This community feature is especially important for seniors' emotional health, as it helps them overcome loneliness and retain a positive attitude toward life. Regular attendance at group sessions can also give accountability, making it easier to maintain consistency in practice.

Consistency is crucial to realizing the full potential of somatic exercises. Seniors who commit to regular practice can experience significant improvements in mobility, pain alleviation, and emotional well-being. These advantages are not only ephemeral; they reinforce one another, laying the groundwork for long-term health and energy.

Seniors can rediscover the joy of movement, reclaim their independence, and develop a stronger connection to their bodies by engaging in mindful repetition. Consistency is more than a habit; it is a road to success at any age.

CONCLUSION

As we near the end of this journey through somatic workouts developed for seniors, it is vital to consider the great potential that somatic movement has for increasing quality of life. The gentle, thoughtful exercises in this book provide more than simply physical advantages; they are a comprehensive approach to pain alleviation, stress reduction, and mental well-being. The work done in this place is more than just physical movement; it's about strengthening the bond between mind, body, and soul. This relationship enables us to age gracefully, mitigate the effects of chronic pain, and regain flexibility and mobility that we may have thought were lost forever.

Somatic movement is a very effective tool for reclaiming our bodies and brains. Somatic activities differ from standard workouts in that they emphasize the natural flow of movement, conscious awareness, and the release of tension and stress rather than strength and endurance through repetitive, high-impact exercises. These exercises are great for seniors who may be experiencing joint stiffness, balance difficulties, or pain while simultaneously wishing to preserve or recover vitality and mobility.

Pain, particularly chronic pain, can drastically limit our capacity to enjoy daily activities while also causing feelings of frustration, loneliness, and melancholy. Somatic exercises are especially beneficial in addressing these difficulties because they educate the body to release tension, relax tight muscles, and improve posture, all of which can help relieve pain. Seniors can manage and lessen physical discomfort associated with aging by focusing on slow, controlled movements and breathing, allowing them to feel more comfortable in their bodies.

The relationship between somatic movement and pain relief is profoundly entrenched in neuroplasticity, or the brain's ability to reorganize itself in response to experience. Seniors who do somatic exercises educate their nervous system on new movement patterns, diminishing those that have been established over time as a result of injury, bad posture, or compensations for earlier suffering. Over time, this rewiring helps to alleviate pain and improve physical function.

Stress can also be detrimental to our physical and mental health. The mild nature of somatic activities, particularly the emphasis on breathwork, activates the parasympathetic nervous system, facilitating relaxation and mitigating the effects of daily stressors. Somatic movement can provide an anchor for emotional stability for seniors who are experiencing life upheavals such as retirement, loss of loved ones, or health issues. Moving with intention and awareness promotes mental clarity, reduces anxiety, and fosters a sense of peace and relaxation.

As we age, we often lose flexibility and mobility, particularly in the spine, hips, shoulders, and legs. Stiffness in these areas can cause limited range of motion, trouble with daily activities, and even an increased risk of falling. Somatic activities, which focus on slow, conscious movement and gentle stretching, aid elders in regaining flexibility and mobility in a safe and regulated manner.

Throughout the book, you've been introduced to a variety of somatic exercises designed to relieve tension in certain parts of the body, including the neck, back, shoulders, pelvis, and legs. These exercises are intended to gradually increase movement in the joints and muscles, ultimately restoring a complete range of motion. Importantly, somatic techniques allow seniors to move within their limitations, eliminating the risk of overexertion or injury. Seniors who incorporate these exercises into their regular routines can gradually increase their flexibility, resulting in a higher capacity to accomplish daily tasks with ease, less muscle stiffness, and a stronger sense of vitality.

Consistency is a key feature of somatic exercises. While it is normal to experience short-term results after just a few sessions, the actual advantages of somatic movement require consistent practice. Somatic exercises are not intended to provide a quick fix or a "one-time" remedy. They offer a sustainable, long-term approach to health and wellness that can be tailored to any lifestyle.

Seniors can progressively improve their strength, flexibility, and mobility by establishing a daily or weekly regimen that reduces discomfort and stress. The beauty of somatic exercises is their versatility. These exercises can be performed at home, in a chair, or lying down—whichever works best for the individual. For seniors with restricted mobility, even minor motions can have a huge impact on their health and well-being. Additionally, mindfulness and deep breathing can be integrated into various aspects of life to assist manage stress and promote mental wellness.

Creating a routine also motivates elders to stay devoted to their health, promoting a sense of accomplishment and self-care. Somatic exercises, whether practiced for 15 minutes or more each day, can become an essential part of a senior's lifestyle, bringing long-term physical and emotional advantages.

Somatic movement is a lifelong practice that can help seniors as they age. The exercises in this book are adaptable to the changing needs of the body as it evolves. While it may take some time to achieve complete effects, the trip is extremely gratifying. Seniors who engage in somatic activities will feel more connected to their bodies, empowered by their ability to handle pain, stress, and tension, and energized by greater mobility and flexibility.

Seniors who embrace somatic movement not only engage in their physical health but also actively work to improve their mental and emotional well-being. Moving with awareness, breath, and intention is more than simply a physical workout; it is a type of self-care that benefits the entire person.

Finally, somatic workouts provide seniors with a mild, effective, and long-term strategy to maintain or improve their health and well-being. Seniors can minimize pain, relieve tension, and regain mobility and flexibility by emphasizing thoughtful, controlled movements, breathing methods, and emotional awareness. The principles of somatic movement pave the way for seniors to live with greater ease, confidence, and vitality, allowing them to fully appreciate the riches of life, regardless of age.

As you continue on your somatic journey, remember that consistency is crucial. Begin with tiny steps, listen to your body, and enjoy the practice. Over time, you will experience long-term changes in your physical and mental well-being. The advantages of somatic movement are within reach, and by committing to this practice, you can begin a new chapter of health, well-being, and peace of mind.

By including somatic exercises in your daily routine, you can continue to thrive long into your golden years, moving with ease, living with vigor, and enjoying the benefits of a tranquil, balanced lifestyle.